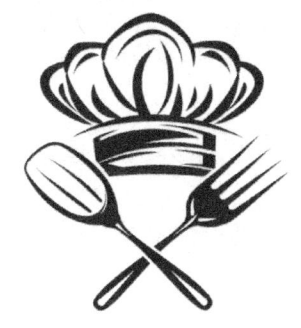

Renal Diet Cookbook for Beginners

Delicious Kidney-Friendly Recipes with Easy
Meal Plans for Managing Health.
Low Sodium, Potassium, and Phosphorus
Meals for a Healthier Life

Sophia Matthews

FREE BONUS!

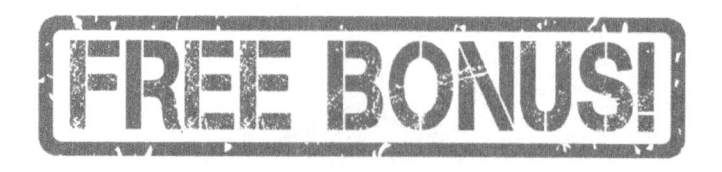

Get Your 6 FREE Exclusive Bonuses Today!

Enjoy a stunning digital version of your cookbook, featuring full-color images for every recipe—something you won't find in the printed book!

🚀 Your FREE Interactive Recipe App

Take your cooking to the next level with features designed just for you:

- ☑ **Interactive Recipes** – Browse a **digital, full-color** version of your cookbook anytime!
- ☑ **Portion Calculator** – Adjust ingredients instantly for any serving size.
- ☑ **Built-in Timers** – Never overcook again with smart reminders.
- ☑ **Personalized Meal Plans** – Weekly menus tailored to your needs.

+ 5 Exclusive Bonus Guides

Unlock additional Renal Diet resources to simplify your meal planning and improve your health.

How to Claim Your Bonuses

**Jump to the End of the Book
Scan the QR Code
Start Exploring Your Exclusive Content!**

Table of Content:

Chapter 1: Welcome to Your Renal Diet Journey 6

Chapter 2: Getting Started with the Renal Diet 9

Chapter 3: Meal Planning Made Easy 13

Chapter 4: Breakfast Recipes 17

1. Oatmeal with Fresh Berries 17
2. Low-Sodium Veggie Omelet 17
3. Cinnamon-Spiced Quinoa 18
4. Banana Pancakes 18
5. Greek Yogurt with Honey and Melon........... 18
6. Avocado Toast with a Twist 19
7. Apple Cinnamon Overnight Oats 19
8. Berry Smoothie... 19
9. Peanut Butter and Banana Toast 20
10. Scrambled Egg Whites with Chives............ 20
11. Almond Butter Smoothie 20
12. Veggie Breakfast Wrap 20
13. Chia Seed Pudding 21
14. Pumpkin Spice Pancakes......................... 21
15. Coconut Yogurt Parfait 21
16. Pear and Ginger Breakfast Bowl 22
17. Sweet Potato Breakfast Hash 22
18. Blueberry Almond Overnight Oats 22
19. Spinach and Mushroom Breakfast Wrap.... 22
20. Raspberry Chia Smoothie........................ 23
21. Quinoa Porridge with Apples 23
22. Vanilla Pear Smoothie............................. 23
23. Lemon Blueberry Pancakes..................... 23
24. Spiced Pear and Oatmeal Muffins............ 24
25. Apple Cinnamon Breakfast Quinoa 24
26. Peach and Cottage Cheese Toast 24
27. Apple Walnut Breakfast Parfait 25
28. Avocado and Tomato Breakfast Salad...... 25
29. Pineapple Coconut Quinoa 25
30. Banana Chia Seed Pudding 26

Chapter 5: Lunch Recipes 27

1. Grilled Chicken Salad with Apple Slices 27
2. Tuna Salad Wrap with Cucumber............... 27
3. Low-Sodium Lentil Soup 28
4. Veggie and Hummus Pita Pocket 28
5. Turkey and Avocado Sandwich.................. 28
6. Quinoa and Black Bean Salad 29
7. Chicken and Spinach Wrap 29
8. Mediterranean Couscous Salad................. 29
9. Shrimp and Avocado Salad....................... 30
10. Pasta Salad with Roasted Vegetables....... 30
11. Chicken Caesar Salad (Lightened Up)........ 31
12. Egg Salad Lettuce Wraps........................ 31
13. Spaghetti Squash with Pesto 31
14. BBQ Tofu Salad 32
15. Turkey and Sweet Potato Bowl................ 32
16. Spiced Chickpea Salad Wrap 32
17. Lentil and Vegetable Soup...................... 33
18. Quinoa and Avocado Salad 33
19. Baked Turkey and Veggie Roll-Ups........... 33
20. Zucchini Noodles with Pesto 34
21. Lemon Chicken and Rice Salad 34
22. Spinach and Feta Stuffed Pita 34
23. Veggie Quinoa Pilaf............................... 34
24. Mediterranean Chickpea Salad............... 35
25. Sweet Potato and Black Bean Tacos 35
26. Turkey Avocado Lettuce Wraps 35
27. Grilled Vegetable Panini 36
28. Shrimp and Cucumber Salad 36
29. Lentil and Quinoa Stuffed Peppers........... 36
30. Greek Yogurt Chicken Salad 36

Chapter 6: Dinner Recipes 38

1. Baked Lemon Herb Chicken...................... 38
2. Grilled Salmon with Dill Sauce 38
3. Grilled Salmon with Avocado Salsa 39
4. Vegetarian Stir-Fry with Tofu 39
5. Baked Cod with Lemon and Garlic 39
6. Turkey Meatballs with Zucchini Noodles......40
7. Quinoa-Stuffed Portobello Mushrooms 40
8. Garlic Shrimp with Asparagus 41
9. Balsamic-Glazed Chicken with Brussels Sprouts 41
10. Turkey Chili 41
11. Baked Eggplant Parmesan 42
12. Lemon Garlic Shrimp Pasta.....................42
13. Roasted Chicken and Vegetables............42
14. Grilled Vegetable Skewers 43
15. Slow-Cooked Beef Stew 43
16. Herb-Crusted Tilapia 43
17. Lemon Herb Chicken with Asparagus 44
18. Vegetable Lentil Stir-Fry......................... 44
19. Garlic Shrimp with Spinach 44
20. Balsamic Glazed Chicken with Roasted Vegetables 45
21. Herb-Roasted Salmon with Carrots 45

22. Turkey and Quinoa Stuffed Bell Peppers 45
23. Roasted Eggplant and Tomato Stew 46
24. Chicken and Cauliflower Rice Stir-Fry...... 46
25. Coconut Curry with Vegetables 46
26. Moroccan-Spiced Chickpea Stew............ 47
27. Lemon Baked Cod with Asparagus 47
28. Cauliflower and Spinach Curry................. 47
29. Baked Chicken with Lemon and Thyme..... 48
30. Eggplant and Tomato Casserole............. 48

Chapter 7: Snack Recipes 50
1. Apple Slices with Almond Butter 50
2. Cucumber and Hummus Bites 50
3. Rice Cakes with Avocado Spread............... 50
4. Fresh Veggies with Yogurt Dip..................... 51
5. Homemade Popcorn 51
6. Mixed Berries with Mint 51
7. Peanut Butter Banana Bites 52
8. Hard-Boiled Egg with Paprika 52
9. Almonds and Raisins Mix 52
10. Smoothie with Spinach and Pineapple 52
11. Sliced Bell Peppers with Guacamole 53
12. Yogurt with Honey and Berries................... 53
13. Carrot and Celery Sticks with Peanut Butter... 53
14. Baked Kale Chips 53
15. Carrot and Hummus Roll-Ups 54
16. Blueberry Almond Bites............................... 54
17. Spiced Apple Chips...................................... 54
18. Cherry Tomato and Mozzarella Skewers.... 54
19. Edamame with Lemon Zest 55
20. Frozen Grapes 55
21. Roasted Bell Pepper Slices 55
22. Banana Oat Bites... 55
23. Pear and Cheese Bites 56
24. Tomato Basil Bruschetta 56
25. Radish Chips 56
26. Zucchini Fries 56
27. Cucumber Mint Salad 57
28. Baked Sweet Potato Slices 57

Chapter 8: Dessert Recipes.......................58
1. Berry Parfait... 58
2. Cinnamon Baked Apples 58
3. Banana Oat Cookies 58
4. Lemon Sorbet... 59
5. Chocolate Chia Pudding 59
6. Baked Pears with Honey 59
7. Coconut Macaroons 60
8. Vanilla Almond Milk Pudding 60
9. Raspberry Sorbet.. 60
10. Strawberry Banana Ice Cream 61
11. Peach Crisp.. 61

12. Blueberry Muffins 61
13. Chocolate-Dipped Strawberries................ 62
14. Vanilla Rice Pudding.................................... 62
15. Mango Sorbet 62
16. Roasted Chickpeas 63
17. Cucumber Slices with Feta and Dill 63
18. Apple Nachos 63
19. Veggie Sticks with Hummus 63
20. Spiced Pumpkin Seeds 64
21. Watermelon and Mint Skewers 64
22. Cottage Cheese with Pineapple 64
23. Avocado Deviled Eggs 64
24. Pear and Walnut Bites................................. 65
25. Celery Sticks with Almond Butter.............. 65
26. Mini Rice Cakes with Tomato and Basil 65
27. Frozen Banana Bites 65
28. Mango Salsa with Lime 66
29. Radish and Cucumber Salad Cups...........66
30. Cottage Cheese and Melon Bowl............66

Chapter 9: Kidney-Friendly Drinks, Smoothies, and Juices 68
1. Lemon Mint Water 68
2. Iced Herbal Tea..68
3. Berry Smoothie..69
4. Cucumber Cooler..69
5. Apple Ginger Tea...69
6. Coconut Water Refresher........................... 70
7. Peach Iced Tea... 70
8. Cinnamon Apple Water............................... 70
9. Watermelon Cooler 71
10 Tropical Green Smoothie 71
11. Warm Vanilla Almond Milk.......................... 71
12. Berry Delight Smoothie 71
13. Cucumber Mint Cooler................................ 72
14. Apple Ginger Smoothie 72
15. Creamy Peach Smoothie 72
16. Strawberry Basil Refresher........................ 72
17. Pineapple Coconut Smoothie....................73
18. Watermelon Lime Cooler.............................73
19. Banana Almond Smoothie..........................73
20. Honeydew Mint Juice...................................73
21. Papaya Ginger Smoothie 74
22. Kiwi Spinach Smoothie 74
23. Blueberry Coconut Juice 74
24. Carrot Apple Juice...................................... 74
25. Mango Lime Smoothie 75
26. Pineapple Celery Juice 75
27. Green Melon Smoothie................................75
28. Raspberry Lemonade Smoothie 75
29. Orange Carrot Smoothie 76
30. Pear Vanilla Smoothie.................................76
31. Peach Mango Smoothie..............................76

32. Grape Apple Juice 76
33. Melon Mint Refresher 77

Chapter 10: Special Occasions and Holiday Recipes 78
1. Roast Turkey with Herb Rub 78
2. Sweet Potato Mash (Low-Potassium) 78
3. Green Bean Casserole 79
4. Cranberry Sauce (Low-Sugar) 79
5. Apple and Pear Crumble 79
6. Herb-Crusted Pork Tenderloin 80
7. Pumpkin Pie (Low-Sugar) 80
8. Garlic Mashed Cauliflower 80
9. Holiday Spiced Pears 81
10. Festive Roasted Brussels Sprouts 81
11. Holiday Apple Cider Punch 81
12. Light Herb Stuffing 81
13. Carrot and Parsnip Mash 82
14. No-Bake Holiday Chocolate Bites 82

Chapter 11: 30-Day Meal Plan 83

Chapter 12: Practical Tips for Living a Kidney-Friendly Lifestyle 87

Chapter 13: Dining Out on a Renal Diet 90

Chapter 14: Conclusion and Next Steps 92

Glossary of Key Terms 94

Get your free bonuses 97

Chapter 1: Welcome to Your Renal Diet Journey

Welcome to the Renal Diet Journey

Hey there, kidney warrior! 🎉 First of all, let's take a moment to give you a well-deserved round of applause for taking this step toward better health. Deciding to embrace a renal diet is no small feat, and I'm thrilled to be your guide on this journey. Whether you're here because of a recent diagnosis, or you're just looking to up your kidney care game, you've come to the right place.

You might be feeling a mix of emotions right now—curiosity, concern, maybe even a little bit of overwhelm. And that's totally okay. Think of this book as your trusty sidekick, here to walk with you every step of the way. We're going to take the mystery out of renal dieting, sprinkle in some tasty recipes, and make sure that your kidneys get all the love they need. You're not alone in this, and with the right tools and mindset, you're going to crush it!

This isn't just a diet; it's a lifestyle makeover that's all about boosting your health and happiness. We're not talking about giving up your favorite foods or spending hours slaving away in the kitchen. Nope! We're about to explore a world where healthy, kidney-friendly eating is delicious, easy, and totally doable.

So, grab your favorite beverage, get comfy, and let's dive in. Your journey to a healthier, happier life starts right here, right now.

Understanding Kidney Health: A Simple Guide

Alright, let's break it down. Your kidneys are like the VIP bouncers at the club that is your body. They keep the place running smoothly by filtering out the riffraff—excess waste, toxins, and fluids—so everything stays in tip-top shape. But when your kidneys start feeling the pressure, they need a little extra support to keep things flowing (literally).

Think of your renal diet as the best assistant your kidneys could ever ask for. By carefully choosing what goes on your plate, you're lightening their load and helping them keep up the good work. It's like giving your kidneys a well-deserved spa day, every day.

Now, you might be wondering, "What exactly is a renal diet, and why do I need one?" Great question! A renal diet focuses on managing your intake of key minerals like sodium, potassium, and phosphorus. These guys are crucial for your body, but when your kidneys aren't functioning at full power, they can start to cause trouble if not kept in check.

Sodium, for instance, loves to hang on to water, which can lead to swelling and high blood pressure—things we definitely want to avoid. Potassium, while important for muscle function, can be a bit of a double-edged sword if it builds up too much. And phosphorus? It's great for bones, but too much of it can lead to serious problems when your kidneys can't filter it out efficiently.

This book is going to help you navigate these nutritional waters with ease. You'll learn how to make smart food choices that support your kidney health, all while enjoying meals that are anything but boring. We're talking about delicious, satisfying recipes that are low in sodium, potassium, and phosphorus, but high in flavor and fun.

So, if you're ready to turn your kitchen into a kidney-friendly oasis, let's get started. Your kidneys (and taste buds) are in for a treat!

How This Cookbook Can Help You

Now, let's get into the nitty-gritty of why this cookbook is your new best friend. Picture this: you're standing in the kitchen, staring at your pantry, and wondering, "What on earth am I going to eat that won't upset my kidneys?" That's where this book comes in.

Here's what you'll find inside:

- **A Treasure Trove of Recipes:** We've packed this book with 2000 days' worth of recipes that are tailor-made for a renal diet. From breakfast to dinner, snacks to desserts, we've got something for every craving. And the best part? These recipes are easy to make and even easier to enjoy.
- **A Foolproof 100-Day Meal Plan:** Let's face it—planning meals can be a chore, especially when you're juggling dietary restrictions. That's why we've done the heavy lifting for you with a detailed 100-day meal plan. Just follow along, and you'll have a kidney-friendly menu ready to go without the stress.
- **Nutritional Know-How:** We're not just handing you recipes; we're giving you the tools to understand the "why" behind your food choices. You'll get a crash course in reading nutrition labels, learning how to balance your meals, and making substitutions that keep your diet on track.
- **Tips for Real Life:** This book isn't just about what happens in your kitchen. We're also covering the real-world stuff, like how to make smart choices when you're dining out, how to handle social situations where food is involved, and even how to indulge a little during the holidays without going off the rails.

So why does this matter? Because living with kidney disease shouldn't mean giving up the joy of eating. This cookbook is designed to empower you with knowledge, inspire you with tasty recipes, and help you feel confident in your ability to manage your health. You've got this!

Tips for Success on a Renal Diet

Ready to set yourself up for success? Here are some tried-and-true tips that will make sticking to your renal diet a piece of cake (a kidney-friendly one, of course):

1. **Prep Like a Pro:** The key to staying on track is preparation. Take advantage of the meal plans and shopping lists in this book. Spend a little time each week planning out your meals, so you're not caught off guard when hunger strikes.
2. **Mix Things Up:** Variety is the spice of life—and of your renal diet. Don't be afraid to experiment with new recipes, try different herbs and spices, and explore the full range of kidney-friendly foods available to you. Keeping your diet exciting will make it easier to stick with.
3. **Hydrate Wisely:** Water is essential, but when you're managing kidney issues, you need to be mindful of your fluid intake. This book will guide you on how much you should be drinking and what kinds of fluids are best for you.
4. **Become a Label Detective:** One of the most important skills you can develop is the ability to read and understand food labels. Look out for hidden sources of sodium, potassium, and phosphorus. Once you get the hang of it, you'll feel like a nutrition ninja!

5. **Celebrate Small Wins:** It's important to recognize and celebrate your progress, no matter how small. Whether it's mastering a new recipe, sticking to your meal plan for a week, or just making it through a tough day without giving in to temptation, give yourself a pat on the back. Every victory counts.

6. **Stay Positive:** Let's keep it real—there will be days when sticking to your diet feels like a challenge. But remember, you're doing this for your health, and every positive choice you make is a step towards feeling better and living your best life.

7. **Seek Support:** Don't go it alone. Whether it's joining a community of people who are also managing kidney health, talking to a dietitian, or simply sharing your journey with friends and family, having a support system can make all the difference.

8. **Be Kind to Yourself:** Finally, remember that nobody's perfect. If you slip up, don't beat yourself up about it. Just get back on track with your next meal and keep moving forward. This is a journey, and every step you take is a step towards better health.

With these tips in your toolkit, you're ready to take on the renal diet like a champ. Remember, this isn't about perfection—it's about progress. So take a deep breath, stay positive, and let's get cooking! Your kidneys are going to love the delicious journey you're about to embark on.

Chapter 2: Getting Started with the Renal Diet

What is a Renal Diet?

Alright, so let's dive into the heart of the matter—what exactly is a renal diet, and why is it so important for your kidneys? Imagine your kidneys as the hardworking heroes in your body's factory, processing everything you eat and drink. When they're healthy, they do their job without breaking a sweat, but when they're under pressure, they need a little extra help to keep things running smoothly.

A renal diet is like giving your kidneys the VIP treatment they deserve. It's a way of eating that's designed to reduce the workload on your kidneys by carefully controlling certain nutrients—namely sodium, potassium, and phosphorus. These are the three amigos that can either be your best friends or your worst enemies, depending on how much of them you consume.

- **Sodium**: This guy is everywhere—seriously, he's in almost everything! But too much sodium can cause your body to hold onto water, leading to high blood pressure and making your kidneys work overtime. On a renal diet, you'll be cutting back on sodium to help keep your blood pressure in check and reduce the strain on your kidneys.
- **Potassium**: Potassium is crucial for keeping your heart and muscles working properly, but when your kidneys aren't functioning at full speed, too much potassium can build up in your blood. This can lead to some pretty serious issues, like irregular heartbeats. That's why a renal diet keeps potassium intake at a safe level.
- **Phosphorus**: Phosphorus is another essential nutrient, especially for your bones and teeth, but when your kidneys can't filter it out properly, it can cause your bones to become weak and brittle. Plus, it can lead to itchy skin and joint pain. On a renal diet, you'll learn to manage phosphorus intake to keep everything balanced.

The goal of a renal diet is to keep these nutrients in check so your kidneys can focus on what they do best—keeping your body healthy. And the best part? With the right recipes and meal plans, you won't feel deprived or restricted. Instead, you'll discover a whole new world of flavors and foods that are as good for your taste buds as they are for your kidneys.

The Role of Sodium, Potassium, and Phosphorus

Now that you've met the big three—sodium, potassium, and phosphorus—let's take a closer look at their roles and why managing them is crucial for kidney health.

1. Sodium: The Sneaky Saboteur

- Sodium's main job is to help balance fluids in your body, but too much of it can throw things out of whack. On a renal diet, your mission is to become a sodium sleuth, finding and reducing hidden sources of sodium in your food. This means choosing fresh, whole foods over processed ones and getting creative with herbs and spices to add flavor without the salt.

2. Potassium: The Muscle Mover

- Potassium is a key player in keeping your muscles, including your heart, working smoothly. But when your kidneys are struggling, it's easy for potassium levels to spike. That's why your renal diet will include foods that are low in potassium but still packed with nutrients. You'll also learn some sneaky ways to reduce potassium in foods, like soaking potatoes before cooking them.

3. Phosphorus: The Bone Builder

- Phosphorus is vital for strong bones and teeth, but it's a bit of a double-edged sword when it comes to kidney health. On a renal diet, you'll be swapping out high-phosphorus foods like dairy and certain meats for kidney-friendly alternatives. You'll also discover some delicious ways to get the calcium you need without the extra phosphorus.

Managing these nutrients might sound tricky at first, but with a little practice, it'll become second nature. And remember, you're not alone in this—this book is here to guide you every step of the way, with recipes and tips that make kidney-friendly eating a breeze.

Essential Nutritional Guidelines for Kidney Health

Alright, so we've talked about what you need to avoid, but what about what you should be eating? Here's a quick rundown of the nutritional guidelines that will help you keep your kidneys in top shape:

- **Focus on Fresh, Whole Foods**: Processed foods are often loaded with sodium, phosphorus, and other additives that can be tough on your kidneys. Stick to fresh fruits, vegetables, lean meats, and whole grains whenever possible.
- **Watch Your Portions**: Even kidney-friendly foods can become a problem if you eat too much of them. Keep an eye on portion sizes, and try to balance your plate with a variety of foods.
- **Stay Hydrated**: Water is essential for helping your kidneys filter waste, but if you're on a fluid restriction, you'll need to be mindful of how much you drink. Your doctor or dietitian can help you figure out the right amount of fluids for your needs.
- **Protein Control**: While protein is important for building and repairing tissues, too much of it can be hard on your kidneys. On a renal diet, you'll want to choose high-quality protein sources like lean meats, fish, eggs, and plant-based proteins, but in moderation.
- **Limit Dairy**: Dairy products are high in phosphorus and potassium, so you'll need to limit your intake. Don't worry, though—there are plenty of delicious non-dairy alternatives that are easy on your kidneys.
- **Be Cautious with Carbs**: Carbohydrates can be a tricky part of a renal diet, especially if you're also managing diabetes. Focus on whole grains and low-sugar options, and avoid refined carbs like white bread and sugary snacks.
- **Mind Your Fat Intake**: Healthy fats are important for overall health, but too much of the wrong kind can lead to weight gain and other health issues. Stick to healthy fats like olive oil, avocado, and nuts, but remember to watch your portions.

These guidelines might seem overwhelming at first, but don't worry—we're going to break it all down in the chapters ahead. By the end of this book, you'll have a solid understanding of how to nourish your body while giving your kidneys the support they need.

Creating a Renal-Friendly Kitchen: Tools and Ingredients

So, you're ready to take charge of your diet—awesome! The first step is to set up your kitchen for success. Having the right tools and ingredients on hand can make all the difference when it comes to sticking to your renal diet. Let's take a look at what you'll need:

Kitchen Essentials

- **Sharp Knives**: A good set of sharp knives makes chopping and prepping your ingredients a breeze.
- **Cutting Boards**: Have separate cutting boards for meat and vegetables to avoid cross-contamination.
- **Measuring Cups and Spoons**: Portion control is key on a renal diet, so measuring tools are a must.
- **Food Scale**: A food scale can help you weigh out portions, especially for meats and other high-protein foods.
- **Non-Stick Pans**: Non-stick pans make cooking with less oil easier, which is great for keeping your fat intake in check.
- **Blender or Food Processor**: Perfect for making kidney-friendly smoothies, soups, and sauces.

Pantry Staples

- **Herbs and Spices**: Ditch the salt and stock up on herbs and spices like basil, thyme, garlic, and onion powder. These will become your go-to flavor boosters.
- **Low-Sodium Broth**: A great base for soups and stews without the extra sodium.
- **Olive Oil**: A healthy fat that's perfect for cooking and dressings.
- **Whole Grains**: Brown rice, quinoa, and whole wheat pasta are excellent choices for your renal diet.
- **Canned Beans (No Salt Added)**: A good source of protein and fiber, just be sure to rinse them well.
- **Non-Dairy Milk**: Almond milk, rice milk, and coconut milk are good alternatives to dairy.

Fridge and Freezer Must-Haves

- **Fresh Vegetables**: Leafy greens, bell peppers, cucumbers, and carrots should be staples in your fridge.
- **Lean Proteins**: Chicken breast, turkey, fish, and eggs are great protein options.
- **Fresh Fruits**: Apples, berries, and grapes are delicious, low-potassium options.
- **Frozen Vegetables**: Keep a stash of frozen veggies for quick and easy meal prep.
- **Low-Sodium Condiments**: Look for low-sodium ketchup, mustard, and salad dressings.

Setting up your kitchen with these essentials will make it easier to prepare kidney-friendly meals without the stress. Plus, having a well-stocked pantry and fridge means you'll always have the ingredients you need to whip up something delicious.

Shopping Tips for a Renal Diet

Grocery shopping on a renal diet doesn't have to be a daunting task. With a little preparation and these handy tips, you'll be navigating the aisles like a pro:

- **Make a List**: Before you head to the store, plan your meals for the week and make a shopping list. This will help you stay focused and avoid impulse buys that might not fit your diet.
- **Shop the Perimeter**: The perimeter of the store is where you'll find fresh produce, lean proteins, and whole grains. These are the staples of your renal diet, so spend most of your time here.

- **Read Labels**: Become a label-reading ninja. Look for low-sodium options and check the serving size to make sure you're not getting more sodium, potassium, or phosphorus than you bargained for.
- **Choose Fresh Over Processed**: Fresh foods are almost always better for your kidneys than processed ones. If you do buy packaged foods, look for those with the fewest ingredients.
- **Avoid the Snack Aisle**: Prepackaged snacks are often loaded with sodium, sugar, and unhealthy fats. Instead, stock up on kidney-friendly snacks like fresh fruit, unsalted nuts, and homemade popcorn.
- **Don't Be Afraid to Ask**: If you're unsure about a product or need help finding low-sodium options, don't hesitate to ask a store employee. Many stores also have dietitians who can offer guidance.
- **Buy in Bulk**: If you find a good deal on renal-friendly staples, buy in bulk. Just make sure to store everything properly so it stays fresh.

By following these shopping tips, you'll be able to fill your cart with foods that support your kidney health without feeling overwhelmed.

By the end of this chapter, you should feel more confident about starting your renal diet journey. Armed with the knowledge of what to eat, how to manage key nutrients, and how to set up your kitchen, you're well on your way to making healthy, kidney-friendly eating a part of your daily routine.

Let's keep this momentum going as we dive into the delicious recipes and meal plans that will make your renal diet both manageable and enjoyable.

Chapter 3: Meal Planning Made Easy

The 100-Day Meal Plan: A Step-by-Step Guide

So you've decided to dive into the renal diet, but now you might be wondering, "What's for dinner?" Well, wonder no more! We've got you covered with a 100-day meal plan that takes all the guesswork out of what to eat. This plan is designed to help you transition smoothly into a kidney-friendly lifestyle without feeling overwhelmed.

Think of this meal plan as your personal roadmap. It's structured to provide balance, variety, and all the nutrients your body needs, while also keeping your kidneys in mind. Each day's menu includes breakfast, lunch, dinner, and snacks, so you're never left guessing.

Here's how to make the most of your 100-day meal plan:

- **Start with the Basics**: The first few weeks are all about getting comfortable with new foods and cooking techniques. We'll introduce you to kidney-friendly staples, so you can build a solid foundation.
- **Introduce Variety**: As you move through the plan, you'll notice a gradual introduction of new recipes and flavors. This is to keep your meals exciting and ensure you're not getting bored with the same dishes every day.
- **Adjust as Needed**: Everyone's dietary needs are a bit different, especially when it comes to managing kidney health. Feel free to swap out meals or ingredients as needed to suit your taste and nutritional needs. This plan is flexible!
- **Prep Ahead**: Each week, take some time to review the upcoming meals and prepare anything you can in advance. Chopping veggies, marinating proteins, or even cooking a batch of rice can save you time and stress during busy weekdays.
- **Stay Hydrated**: Your meal plan will also include recommendations for daily fluid intake. Remember, hydration is key, but you'll need to manage your fluid intake based on your specific needs.
- **Monitor Your Progress**: As you follow the meal plan, pay attention to how you're feeling. If something isn't working for you, don't be afraid to tweak the plan. This is your journey, and it's important to listen to your body.

By following this meal plan, you'll not only be eating delicious, kidney-friendly meals, but you'll also be forming habits that will serve you well for years to come. Ready to see what's on the menu? Let's dive in!

How to Customize Your Meal Plan

While the 100-day meal plan is a great starting point, it's important to remember that flexibility is key. Everyone has different tastes, schedules, and nutritional needs, so feel free to make adjustments that work for you.

Here's how you can customize your meal plan:

- **Swap Out Proteins**: If you're not a fan of chicken but love fish, go ahead and make the swap. Just be mindful of portion sizes and cooking methods to keep everything kidney-friendly.
- **Adjust Portions**: Depending on your stage of kidney disease and your overall health, you might need to adjust portion sizes. For example, if you need to limit protein, try reducing the portion size of meat or fish and increasing your servings of vegetables.

- **Mix and Match**: Don't be afraid to mix and match meals from different days. If you really love a particular recipe, you can repeat it during the week. The goal is to make the meal plan work for you, not the other way around.
- **Incorporate Seasonal Ingredients:** Eating seasonally can be a great way to enjoy fresh, flavorful produce. Feel free to swap out vegetables or fruits based on what's in season in your area.
- **Accommodate Your Schedule**: If you're busy during the week, consider prepping meals on the weekend. Double up on recipes that store well, like soups or casseroles, so you have leftovers ready to go when time is tight.
- **Consider Your Fluid Needs**: Depending on your fluid restrictions, you may need to adjust the types of drinks or the amount of soup and other liquid-rich foods you consume. Your doctor or dietitian can help you figure out what's best.

Customizing your meal plan allows you to make the most of this diet without feeling restricted. It's all about finding the balance that keeps your kidneys happy and your taste buds satisfied.

Reading Nutrition Labels: What to Look For

One of the most empowering skills you can develop on a renal diet is learning how to read nutrition labels like a pro. This will help you make informed choices at the grocery store and ensure that what you're eating supports your kidney health.

Here's what to focus on when reading labels:

Serving Size: Always check the serving size first. All the nutrition information on the label is based on this amount, so if you eat more or less, you'll need to adjust the numbers accordingly.

Sodium Content: Sodium is a biggie. Aim for foods that have less than 140 mg of sodium per serving, which is considered low sodium. Avoid products with more than 300 mg per serving, as these can quickly add up and strain your kidneys.

Potassium Levels: Not all labels list potassium, but when they do, aim for lower amounts. Ideally, look for foods with less than 200 mg of potassium per serving.

Phosphorus Additives: Phosphorus isn't always listed on nutrition labels, but it's often hidden in ingredients like "phosphate" or "phosphoric acid." Try to avoid these additives, as they can be absorbed more easily by your body than natural phosphorus found in foods.

Protein Content: Depending on your dietary needs, you might need to keep an eye on protein. Look for products that offer quality protein without going overboard—typically around 7-10 grams per serving.

Added Sugars: Many processed foods contain added sugars, which can lead to weight gain and other health issues. Look for foods with little to no added sugars, or opt for natural sweeteners when possible.

Calcium and Vitamin D: While these nutrients are important, if you're trying to limit phosphorus, you might want to be cautious with fortified foods. Choose natural sources when possible, or discuss supplementation with your healthcare provider.

By mastering the art of label reading, you'll be able to make smarter food choices that align with your renal diet. This is a powerful tool in your journey to better health, giving you the confidence to navigate any grocery aisle with ease.

Managing Fluid Intake: What You Need to Know

For many people with kidney issues, managing fluid intake is just as important as managing what you eat. While staying hydrated is crucial, too much fluid can put a strain on your kidneys and lead to complications like swelling and high blood pressure.

Here's how to manage your fluid intake effectively:

Know Your Limit: Your doctor or dietitian will give you a recommended daily fluid limit. This includes not just what you drink, but also the fluids in foods like soups, fruits, and even some vegetables.

Track Your Fluids: Keep a daily log of how much fluid you're consuming. This can help you stay within your limits and avoid accidentally overdoing it.

Choose Your Drinks Wisely: Water is usually the best choice, but if you're looking for variety, opt for kidney-friendly options like low-sodium broths or herbal teas. Avoid sugary drinks, sodas, and those high in sodium or potassium.

Watch Out for Hidden Fluids: Foods like watermelon, grapes, oranges, and lettuce contain a lot of water, so factor these into your daily fluid count.

Ice Chips Are Your Friend: If you're feeling thirsty but need to limit fluids, sucking on ice chips can help keep your mouth moist without adding too much liquid.

Season with Caution: Certain seasonings, like salt substitutes, can contain high levels of potassium, which might lead to fluid retention. Stick to herbs and spices that are low in sodium and potassium instead.

Stay Cool: In hot weather, your fluid needs might change. Make sure to adjust your intake accordingly, and consult your healthcare provider if you're unsure.

By staying mindful of your fluid intake and making informed choices, you can keep your kidneys functioning as well as possible and avoid the complications that come with fluid overload.

Food Substitutions for a Renal Diet

One of the challenges of following a renal diet is finding suitable substitutions for common ingredients that are high in sodium, potassium, or phosphorus. But don't worry—there are plenty of tasty alternatives out there!

Here are some easy swaps to make your favorite recipes kidney-friendly:

Instead of Salt, Try...

- Fresh or dried herbs like basil, thyme, or rosemary
- Spices like garlic powder, onion powder, or black pepper
- Lemon juice or vinegar for a tangy kick

Instead of High-Potassium Vegetables (e.g., Potatoes, Tomatoes), Try...

- Cauliflower or turnips for mash or fries
- Red bell peppers, zucchini, or green beans in sauces or salads

Instead of Dairy Products (High in Phosphorus and Potassium), Try...

- Unsweetened almond milk or rice milk
- Non-dairy cheese made from rice or almond

- Greek yogurt (in moderation) or non-dairy yogurt

Instead of Processed Meats (High in Sodium), Try...

- Fresh, lean cuts of chicken, turkey, or fish
- Homemade burgers or meatloaf with low-sodium seasoning
- Egg whites or tofu for protein-rich, low-sodium options

Instead of Regular Bread (Often High in Sodium and Phosphorus), Try...

- Low-sodium, whole grain bread or pita
- Rice cakes (unsalted) or corn tortillas
- Homemade bread with low-sodium ingredients

Instead of Snack Foods (e.g., Chips, Pretzels), Try...

- Unsalted popcorn or rice cakes
- Fresh veggies with a kidney-friendly dip
- Unsalted nuts or seeds in moderation

Instead of Sugary Desserts, Try...

- Fresh fruit like berries, apples, or grapes
- Homemade fruit sorbet or popsicles
- Low-sugar baked goods using renal-friendly ingredients

These substitutions will allow you to enjoy a wide variety of dishes without compromising your kidney health. Plus, experimenting with new ingredients can be a fun way to discover new favorite foods!

By the end of this chapter, you should feel confident about planning and preparing meals that support your renal diet. Whether you're following the 100-day meal plan or customizing your own, the key is to find what works best for you and your kidneys. Remember, meal planning is not just about following a strict routine—it's about making choices that empower you to live a healthier, happier life.

Chapter 4: Breakfast Recipes

Starting Your Day Right: The Importance of a Healthy Breakfast

They say breakfast is the most important meal of the day, and when you're following a renal diet, this couldn't be more true. A healthy, balanced breakfast sets the tone for your day, giving you the energy you need while keeping your kidneys in mind. Whether you're rushing out the door or enjoying a leisurely morning, the right breakfast can help you start your day on the right foot.

For many people on a renal diet, mornings can feel like a challenge—especially if you're used to grabbing something quick like a bagel or a sugary cereal. But don't worry! This chapter is packed with easy, delicious, and kidney-friendly breakfast recipes that will make your mornings both nutritious and enjoyable.

We're talking about everything from warm, comforting bowls of oatmeal to light and fluffy pancakes, and even protein-packed smoothies that will keep you full and satisfied until lunch. Plus, each recipe is designed to be low in sodium, potassium, and phosphorus, so you can enjoy your meal without worrying about your kidneys.

So, let's get cracking (pun intended) and explore some tasty breakfast options that will have you looking forward to getting out of bed!

30 Kidney-Friendly Breakfast Recipes

1. Oatmeal with Fresh Berries

2 | 5 min | 10 min

Ingredients:

- 1/2 cup rolled oats
- 1 cup water or unsweetened almond milk
- 1/4 cup fresh blueberries
- 1/4 cup fresh raspberries
- 1 tsp honey or maple syrup (optional)

Instructions:

1. In a small pot, bring water or almond milk to a boil.
2. Add oats, reduce heat, and simmer for 5 minutes, stirring occasionally.
3. Once thickened, remove from heat and stir in berries.
4. Drizzle with honey or maple syrup if desired. Serve warm.

Nutritional Information (per serving):

- Calories: 150
- Protein: 5g
- Carbohydrates: 27g
- Sugars: 8g
- Dietary Fiber: 4g
- Fat: 2g
- Sodium: 5mg
- Potassium: 150mg
- Phosphorus: 110mg

2. Low-Sodium Veggie Omelet

1 | 10 min | 5 min

Ingredients:

- 2 large egg whites
- 1/4 cup chopped bell peppers
- 1/4 cup chopped onions
- 1/4 cup chopped spinach
- 1 tbsp olive oil
- Fresh herbs (basil, parsley) to taste

Instructions:

1. Heat olive oil in a non-stick pan over medium heat.
2. Sauté the onions, bell peppers, and spinach until tender.
3. In a bowl, whisk egg whites and pour over the veggies in the pan.
4. Cook until eggs are set, then fold the omelet in half.
5. Sprinkle with fresh herbs and serve.

Nutritional Information (per serving):

- Calories: 90
- Protein: 7g
- Carbohydrates: 4g
- Sugars: 2g
- Dietary Fiber: 1g
- Fat: 5g
- Sodium: 55mg
- Potassium: 210mg
- Phosphorus: 80mg

3. Cinnamon-Spiced Quinoa

2 | 5 min | 10 min

Ingredients:

- 1/2 cup cooked quinoa
- 1/2 cup unsweetened almond milk
- 1 tsp ground cinnamon
- 1 tbsp raisins or dried cranberries (optional)
- 1 tsp honey (optional)

Instructions:

1. In a small pot, combine quinoa and almond milk. Heat over medium until warm.
2. Stir in cinnamon and raisins or cranberries if using.
3. Sweeten with honey if desired and serve warm.

Nutritional Information (per serving):

- Calories: 130
- Protein: 4g
- Carbohydrates: 22g
- Sugars: 6g
- Dietary Fiber: 3g
- Fat: 2g
- Sodium: 15mg
- Potassium: 180mg
- Phosphorus: 100mg

4. Banana Pancakes

2 | 10 min | 15 min

Ingredients:

- 1 ripe banana, mashed
- 1/2 cup rolled oats
- 1/4 cup unsweetened almond milk
- 1/4 tsp baking powder
- 1 egg white
- 1 tsp vanilla extract

Instructions:

1. In a bowl, combine all ingredients and mix until smooth.
2. Heat a non-stick pan over medium heat and lightly grease.
3. Pour batter into the pan to form small pancakes.
4. Cook until bubbles form on the surface, then flip and cook until golden.
5. Serve with fresh berries or a drizzle of honey.

Nutritional Information (per serving):

- Calories: 170
- Protein: 6g
- Carbohydrates: 30g
- Sugars: 9g
- Dietary Fiber: 4g
- Fat: 3g
- Sodium: 50mg
- Potassium: 200mg
- Phosphorus: 120mg

5. Greek Yogurt with Honey and Melon

1 | 5 min | 0 min

Ingredients:

- 1/2 cup plain Greek yogurt
- 1/4 cup diced honeydew melon
- 1/4 cup diced cantaloupe
- 1 tsp honey
- Fresh mint leaves (optional)

Instructions:

1. Spoon Greek yogurt into a bowl.
2. Top with diced melon and drizzle with honey.

3. Garnish with fresh mint leaves if desired. Serve chilled.

Nutritional Information (per serving):

- Calories: 120
- Protein: 10g
- Carbohydrates: 14g
- Sugars: 11g
- Dietary Fiber: 1g
- Fat: 2g
- Sodium: 55mg
- Potassium: 180mg
- Phosphorus: 150mg

6. Avocado Toast with a Twist
👥 1 | ⏱ 5 min | 🍽 5 min

Ingredients:

- 1 slice low-sodium whole grain bread
- 1/4 ripe avocado, mashed
- 1 slice tomato (optional)
- Fresh lemon juice
- Ground black pepper
- Fresh herbs (cilantro, parsley) to taste

Instructions:

1. Toast the bread to your desired level of crispiness.
2. Spread mashed avocado on top.
3. Add a slice of tomato if using, and squeeze fresh lemon juice over the top.
4. Season with black pepper and herbs.

Nutritional Information (per serving):

- Calories: 180
- Protein: 4g
- Carbohydrates: 22g
- Sugars: 2g
- Dietary Fiber: 7g
- Fat: 10g
- Sodium: 70mg
- Potassium: 350mg
- Phosphorus: 120mg

7. Apple Cinnamon Overnight Oats
👥 2 | ⏱ 5 min | 🍽 0 min (overnight)

Ingredients:

- 1/2 cup rolled oats
- 1/2 cup unsweetened almond milk
- 1/4 cup grated apple
- 1/2 tsp ground cinnamon
- 1 tbsp chopped walnuts (optional)

Instructions:

1. Combine all ingredients in a mason jar or bowl.
2. Stir well, cover, and refrigerate overnight.
3. In the morning, stir and enjoy cold or heat if preferred.

Nutritional Information (per serving):

- Calories: 160
- Protein: 4g
- Carbohydrates: 30g
- Sugars: 10g
- Dietary Fiber: 4g
- Fat: 3g
- Sodium: 10mg
- Potassium: 190mg
- Phosphorus: 130mg

8. Berry Smoothie
👥 1 | ⏱ 5 min | 🍽 0 min

Ingredients:

- 1/2 cup frozen mixed berries
- 1/2 banana
- 1/2 cup unsweetened almond milk
- 1 tbsp ground flaxseed
- 1 tsp honey (optional)

Instructions:

1. Combine all ingredients in a blender.
2. Blend until smooth.
3. Pour into a glass and enjoy.

Nutritional Information (per serving):

- Calories: 140
- Protein: 3g
- Carbohydrates: 28g
- Sugars: 14g
- Dietary Fiber: 5g
- Fat: 3g
- Sodium: 25mg
- Potassium: 250mg
- Phosphorus: 70mg

Chapter 4: Breakfast Recipes

9. Peanut Butter and Banana Toast

👥 1 | ⏱ 5 min | 🍽 5 min

Ingredients:

- 1 slice low-sodium whole grain bread
- 1 tbsp natural peanut butter
- 1/2 banana, sliced
- Ground cinnamon (optional)

Instructions:

1. Toast the bread.
2. Spread peanut butter on the toast.
3. Top with banana slices and sprinkle with cinnamon if desired.

Nutritional Information (per serving):

- Calories: 210
- Protein: 7g
- Carbohydrates: 30g
- Sugars: 12g
- Dietary Fiber: 5g
- Fat: 8g
- Sodium: 90mg
- Potassium: 300mg
- Phosphorus: 140mg

10. Scrambled Egg Whites with Chives

👥 1 | ⏱ 5 min | 🍽 5 min

Ingredients:

- 2 large egg whites
- 1 tbsp unsweetened almond milk
- 1 tbsp chopped chives
- 1 tsp olive oil

Instructions:

1. In a bowl, whisk egg whites and almond milk together.
2. Heat olive oil in a non-stick pan over medium heat.
3. Pour the egg mixture into the pan and cook, stirring gently, until scrambled.
4. Sprinkle with chives and serve warm.

Nutritional Information (per serving):

- Calories: 80
- Protein: 7g
- Carbohydrates: 1g
- Sugars: 0g
- Dietary Fiber: 0g
- Fat: 5g
- Sodium: 55mg
- Potassium: 110mg
- Phosphorus: 85mg

11. Almond Butter Smoothie

👥 1 | ⏱ 5 min | 🍽 0 min

Ingredients:

- 1 tbsp almond butter
- 1/2 banana
- 1/2 cup unsweetened almond milk
- 1 tbsp ground flaxseed
- Ice cubes (optional)

Instructions:

1. Combine all ingredients in a blender.
2. Blend until smooth.
3. Serve immediately.

Nutritional Information (per serving):

- Calories: 180
- Protein: 5g
- Carbohydrates: 20g
- Sugars: 10g
- Dietary Fiber: 4g
- Fat: 9g
- Sodium: 60mg
- Potassium: 260mg
- Phosphorus: 90mg

12. Veggie Breakfast Wrap

👥 1 | ⏱ 10 min | 🍽 5 min

Ingredients:

- 1 low-sodium whole grain tortilla
- 1/4 cup scrambled egg whites
- 1/4 cup chopped bell peppers
- 1/4 cup chopped spinach
- 1 tbsp salsa (optional)

Instructions:

1. Heat the tortilla in a dry pan.
2. Place scrambled egg whites and veggies in the center of the tortilla.

3. Add salsa if desired.
4. Wrap tightly and serve.

Nutritional Information (per serving):

- Calories: 180
- Protein: 10g
- Carbohydrates: 22g
- Sugars: 3g
- Dietary Fiber: 5g
- Fat: 6g
- Sodium: 70mg
- Potassium: 220mg
- Phosphorus: 100mg

13. Chia Seed Pudding

👥 2 | ⏱ 5 min | 🍽 0 min (overnight)

Ingredients:

- 1/4 cup chia seeds
- 1 cup unsweetened almond milk
- 1 tbsp honey or maple syrup
- 1/4 cup fresh berries for topping

Instructions:

1. Mix chia seeds, almond milk, and sweetener in a bowl or jar.
2. Stir well and refrigerate for at least 4 hours or overnight.
3. Top with fresh berries before serving.

Nutritional Information (per serving):

- Calories: 140
- Protein: 4g
- Carbohydrates: 15g
- Sugars: 8g
- Dietary Fiber: 7g
- Fat: 8g
- Sodium: 35mg
- Potassium: 140mg
- Phosphorus: 120mg

14. Pumpkin Spice Pancakes

👥 2 | ⏱ 10 min | 🍽 15 min

Ingredients:

- 1/2 cup rolled oats
- 1/4 cup pumpkin puree
- 1 egg white
- 1/4 cup unsweetened almond milk
- 1/2 tsp pumpkin spice
- 1 tsp vanilla extract

Instructions:

1. Blend all ingredients together until smooth.
2. Heat a non-stick pan over medium heat.
3. Pour the batter to form pancakes and cook until bubbles form.
4. Flip and cook until golden brown. Serve with a drizzle of honey or maple syrup.

Nutritional Information (per serving):

- Calories: 170
- Protein: 6g
- Carbohydrates: 30g
- Sugars: 7g
- Dietary Fiber: 5g
- Fat: 3g
- Sodium: 40mg
- Potassium: 210mg
- Phosphorus: 120mg

15. Coconut Yogurt Parfait

👥 1 | ⏱ 5 min | 🍽 0 min

Ingredients:

- 1/2 cup unsweetened coconut yogurt
- 1/4 cup granola (low-sodium, low-sugar)
- 1/4 cup sliced strawberries
- 1 tbsp shredded coconut (optional)

Instructions:

1. Layer coconut yogurt, granola, and strawberries in a glass.
2. Sprinkle with shredded coconut if desired.
3. Serve immediately.

Nutritional Information (per serving):

- Calories: 150
- Protein: 3g
- Carbohydrates: 22g
- Sugars: 10g
- Dietary Fiber: 4g
- Fat: 6g
- Sodium: 40mg
- Potassium: 120mg
- Phosphorus: 70mg

Chapter 4: Breakfast Recipes

16. Pear and Ginger Breakfast Bowl

👥 1 | ⏱ 5 min | 🍲 0 min

Ingredients:

- 1 ripe pear, chopped
- 1/4 cup rolled oats
- 1/2 cup unsweetened almond milk
- 1/2 tsp fresh ginger, grated
- 1 tsp honey (optional)

Instructions:

1. Combine chopped pear, rolled oats, almond milk, and ginger in a bowl.
2. Drizzle with honey, if desired, and enjoy immediately.

Nutritional Information (per serving):

- Calories: 120
- Protein: 2g
- Carbohydrates: 25g
- Sugars: 12g
- Dietary Fiber: 5g
- Fat: 2g
- Sodium: 15mg
- Potassium: 100mg
- Phosphorus: 35mg

17. Sweet Potato Breakfast Hash

👥 2 | ⏱ 10 min | 🍲 15 min

Ingredients:

- 1 medium sweet potato, peeled and diced
- 1/4 cup red bell pepper, diced
- 1/4 cup onion, diced
- 1 tbsp olive oil
- 1/2 tsp ground cumin
- 1/4 tsp black pepper

Instructions:

1. Heat olive oil in a skillet over medium heat.
2. Add sweet potato, bell pepper, and onion. Sauté for 10-15 minutes, until potatoes are tender.
3. Season with cumin and black pepper before serving.

Nutritional Information (per serving):

- Calories: 150
- Protein: 2g
- Carbohydrates: 29g
- Sugars: 7g
- Dietary Fiber: 4g
- Fat: 5g
- Sodium: 20mg
- Potassium: 300mg
- Phosphorus: 40mg

18. Blueberry Almond Overnight Oats

👥 1 | ⏱ 5 min (Prep) | 🍲 0 min (Overnight Chill)

Ingredients:

- 1/2 cup rolled oats
- 1/2 cup unsweetened almond milk
- 1/4 cup fresh blueberries
- 1 tbsp almond butter
- 1 tsp chia seeds

Instructions:

1. Combine all ingredients in a jar or bowl.
2. Stir well, cover, and refrigerate overnight.
3. In the morning, enjoy cold or warmed up.

Nutritional Information (per serving):

- Calories: 200
- Protein: 6g
- Carbohydrates: 32g
- Sugars: 8g
- Dietary Fiber: 7g
- Fat: 8g
- Sodium: 30mg
- Potassium: 150mg
- Phosphorus: 70mg

19. Spinach and Mushroom Breakfast Wrap

👥 1 | ⏱ 10 min | 🍲 5 min

Ingredients:

- 1 low-sodium whole grain tortilla
- 1/2 cup spinach leaves
- 1/4 cup mushrooms, sliced
- 1 egg white
- 1 tbsp olive oil

Instructions:

1. Heat olive oil in a skillet over medium heat.
2. Sauté spinach and mushrooms until tender.
3. Add egg white and scramble until cooked.
4. Fill the tortilla with the mixture and roll up.

Nutritional Information (per serving):

- Calories: 180
- Protein: 8g
- Carbohydrates: 20g
- Sugars: 2g
- Dietary Fiber: 4g
- Fat: 8g
- Sodium: 80mg
- Potassium: 180mg
- Phosphorus: 100mg

20. Raspberry Chia Smoothie

👥 1 | ⏱ 5 min | 🍽 0 min

Ingredients:

- 1/2 cup raspberries
- 1/2 cup unsweetened almond milk
- 1 tbsp chia seeds
- 1 tsp honey (optional)
- Ice cubes

Instructions:

1. Blend all ingredients until smooth.
2. Serve immediately.

Nutritional Information (per serving):

- Calories: 100
- Protein: 3g
- Carbohydrates: 15g
- Sugars: 8g
- Dietary Fiber: 6g
- Fat: 3g
- Sodium: 15mg
- Potassium: 90mg
- Phosphorus: 50mg

21. Quinoa Porridge with Apples

👥 2 | ⏱ 10 min | 🍽 15 min

Ingredients:

- 1/2 cup cooked quinoa
- 1/2 apple, chopped
- 1/2 cup unsweetened almond milk
- 1 tsp cinnamon
- 1 tsp honey (optional)

Instructions:

1. In a saucepan, combine quinoa, apple, almond milk, and cinnamon.
2. Heat over medium heat until warmed through.
3. Drizzle with honey, if desired, and serve.

Nutritional Information (per serving):

- Calories: 130
- Protein: 4g
- Carbohydrates: 25g
- Sugars: 8g
- Dietary Fiber: 4g
- Fat: 3g
- Sodium: 5mg
- Potassium: 100mg
- Phosphorus: 70mg

22. Vanilla Pear Smoothie

👥 1 | ⏱ 5 min | 🍽 0 min

Ingredients:

- 1 pear, chopped
- 1/2 tsp vanilla extract
- 1/2 cup unsweetened almond milk
- Ice cubes

Instructions:

1. Blend all ingredients until smooth.
2. Serve immediately.

Nutritional Information (per serving):

- Calories: 90
- Protein: 1g
- Carbohydrates: 22g
- Sugars: 14g
- Dietary Fiber: 4g
- Fat: 1g
- Sodium: 10mg
- Potassium: 85mg
- Phosphorus: 15mg

23. Lemon Blueberry Pancakes

👥 2 | ⏱ 10 min | 🍽 10 min

Ingredients:

- 1/2 cup rolled oats

- 1/4 cup unsweetened almond milk
- 1/2 cup fresh blueberries
- 1 egg white
- 1 tsp lemon zest

Instructions:

1. In a bowl, combine oats, almond milk, egg white, and lemon zest.
2. Heat a non-stick pan over medium heat.
3. Pour batter into the pan to form small pancakes.
4. Cook until bubbles form, then flip and cook until golden.
5. Serve with fresh blueberries.

Nutritional Information (per serving):

- Calories: 160
- Protein: 5g
- Carbohydrates: 28g
- Sugars: 7g
- Dietary Fiber: 5g
- Fat: 3g
- Sodium: 40mg
- Potassium: 120mg
- Phosphorus: 60mg

24. Spiced Pear and Oatmeal Muffins

6 | 15 min | 20 min

Ingredients:

- 1 cup rolled oats
- 1/2 cup unsweetened applesauce
- 1/2 cup pear, finely chopped
- 1 egg white
- 1 tsp ground cinnamon
- 1/2 tsp baking powder

Instructions:

1. Preheat oven to 350°F (175°C).
2. In a bowl, mix oats, applesauce, pear, egg white, cinnamon, and baking powder.
3. Spoon batter into muffin tins and bake for 20 minutes.
4. Let cool before serving.

Nutritional Information (per serving):

- Calories: 80
- Protein: 2g
- Carbohydrates: 15g
- Sugars: 5g
- Dietary Fiber: 2g
- Fat: 1g
- Sodium: 15mg
- Potassium: 50mg
- Phosphorus: 25mg

25. Apple Cinnamon Breakfast Quinoa

1 | 5 min | 15 min

Ingredients:

- 1/2 cup cooked quinoa
- 1/2 apple, diced
- 1/2 cup unsweetened almond milk
- 1 tsp ground cinnamon
- 1 tsp honey (optional)

Instructions:

1. In a small pot, combine quinoa, apple, almond milk, and cinnamon.
2. Heat over medium heat until warm and apple is tender.
3. Drizzle with honey, if desired, and serve.

Nutritional Information (per serving):

- Calories: 130
- Protein: 3g
- Carbohydrates: 25g
- Sugars: 10g
- Dietary Fiber: 3g
- Fat: 2g
- Sodium: 5mg
- Potassium: 70mg
- Phosphorus: 40mg

26. Peach and Cottage Cheese Toast

1 | 5 min | 0 min

Ingredients:

- 1 slice low-sodium whole grain bread
- 1/4 cup cottage cheese (low-sodium)
- 1/2 peach, sliced
- 1/4 tsp cinnamon

Instructions:

Chapter 4: Breakfast Recipes

1. Toast the bread to your desired crispness.
2. Spread cottage cheese on the toast and top with peach slices.
3. Sprinkle with cinnamon and serve immediately.

Nutritional Information (per serving):

- Calories: 150
- Protein: 8g
- Carbohydrates: 20g
- Sugars: 7g
- Dietary Fiber: 3g
- Fat: 4g
- Sodium: 120mg
- Potassium: 150mg
- Phosphorus: 90mg

27. Apple Walnut Breakfast Parfait

👥 1 | ⏱ 5 min | 🍳 0 min

Ingredients:

- 1/2 cup plain Greek yogurt (low-sodium)
- 1/2 apple, diced
- 1 tbsp walnuts, chopped
- 1 tsp honey (optional)

Instructions:

1. Layer Greek yogurt, diced apple, and chopped walnuts in a bowl or glass.
2. Drizzle with honey, if desired, and serve immediately.

Nutritional Information (per serving):

- Calories: 160
- Protein: 9g
- Carbohydrates: 22g
- Sugars: 12g
- Dietary Fiber: 3g
- Fat: 5g
- Sodium: 50mg
- Potassium: 140mg
- Phosphorus: 120mg

28. Avocado and Tomato Breakfast Salad

👥 2 | ⏱ 10 min | 🍳 0 min

Ingredients:

- 1/2 avocado, diced
- 1/2 cup cherry tomatoes, halved
- 1 tbsp fresh basil, chopped
- 1 tsp olive oil
- 1 tsp lemon juice

Instructions:

1. Combine avocado, cherry tomatoes, and basil in a bowl.
2. Drizzle with olive oil and lemon juice. Toss gently and serve.

Nutritional Information (per serving):

- Calories: 120
- Protein: 2g
- Carbohydrates: 10g
- Sugars: 2g
- Dietary Fiber: 5g
- Fat: 10g
- Sodium: 5mg
- Potassium: 250mg
- Phosphorus: 30mg

29. Pineapple Coconut Quinoa

👥 2 | ⏱ 10 min | 🍳 15 min

Ingredients:

- 1/2 cup cooked quinoa
- 1/4 cup pineapple chunks
- 1/4 cup unsweetened coconut milk
- 1 tsp honey (optional)

Instructions:

1. In a saucepan, combine quinoa, pineapple, and coconut milk.
2. Heat over medium heat until warm.
3. Drizzle with honey if desired and serve.

Nutritional Information (per serving):

- Calories: 110
- Protein: 3g
- Carbohydrates: 20g
- Sugars: 8g
- Dietary Fiber: 2g
- Fat: 3g
- Sodium: 10mg
- Potassium: 100mg
- Phosphorus: 50mg

30. Banana Chia Seed Pudding

👥 2 | ⏱ 5 min (Prep) | 🍲 0 min (Chill 2 hours)

Ingredients:

- 1 ripe banana, mashed
- 1/4 cup chia seeds
- 1 cup unsweetened almond milk
- 1/2 tsp vanilla extract

Instructions:

1. In a bowl, mix mashed banana, chia seeds, almond milk, and vanilla extract.
2. Cover and refrigerate for at least 2 hours or overnight.
3. Stir well before serving.

Nutritional Information (per serving):

- Calories: 120
- Protein: 4g
- Carbohydrates: 20g
- Sugars: 10g
- Dietary Fiber: 6g
- Fat: 5g
- Sodium: 20mg
- Potassium: 180mg
- Phosphorus: 80mg

Breakfast Tips and Tricks

Making sure you start your day with a balanced, kidney-friendly breakfast is easier than you might think. Here are a few tips to keep in mind:

- **Prep Ahead**: Many of these recipes can be prepared the night before or even a few days in advance. Overnight oats, chia pudding, and smoothies are great grab-and-go options for busy mornings.
- **Balance is Key**: A good breakfast should include a mix of protein, healthy fats, and carbohydrates. This will keep you feeling full and energized throughout the morning.
- **Watch the Add-Ons**: Be mindful of what you're adding to your breakfast. For example, while fruits are healthy, some are higher in potassium. Stick to lower-potassium options like berries and apples.
- **Stay Hydrated**: Don't forget to include a fluid with your meal. Herbal teas, low-sodium broths, or just plain water are excellent choices.

By incorporating these recipes into your morning routine, you'll be starting each day with a meal that not only tastes great but also supports your kidney health. Breakfast doesn't have to be boring or repetitive—instead, it can be a time to enjoy a variety of flavors and set a positive tone for the rest of your day.

Chapter 5: Lunch Recipes

Midday Meals for Sustained Energy

When midday rolls around, you need a meal that's not only filling but also supportive of your kidney health. Lunch is your chance to refuel and recharge, giving you the energy to power through the rest of your day. But let's be real—finding the perfect lunch that fits within the guidelines of a renal diet can sometimes feel like a challenge.

The good news? It doesn't have to be! This chapter is packed with delicious, kidney-friendly lunch recipes that are simple to prepare and full of flavor. Whether you want a satisfying, meaty supper or something light and fresh, these recipes have you covered.

Each recipe is designed to be low in sodium, potassium, and phosphorus, making it easy to enjoy your lunch without worrying about your kidneys. From salads and soups to wraps and more, these lunch options are perfect for busy weekdays or a relaxed weekend meal.

Let's dive into these tasty recipes that will keep you energized and on track with your renal diet goals!

30 Kidney-Friendly Lunch Recipes

1. Grilled Chicken Salad with Apple Slices

👥 2 | ⏱ 10 min | 🍽 10 min

Ingredients:

- 2 boneless, skinless chicken breasts
- 4 cups mixed salad greens
- 1 apple, thinly sliced
- 1/4 cup shredded carrots
- 1/4 cup sliced cucumbers
- 2 tbsp olive oil
- 1 tbsp apple cider vinegar
- Salt-free seasoning blend (optional)

Instructions:

1. Preheat grill to medium-high heat.
2. Season chicken breasts with salt-free seasoning if desired.
3. Grill chicken for 5-6 minutes per side, until fully cooked.
4. In a large bowl, combine salad greens, apple slices, shredded carrots, and sliced cucumbers.
5. Slice grilled chicken and place on top of the salad.
6. Drizzle with olive oil and apple cider vinegar. Toss gently and serve.

Nutritional Information (per serving):

- Calories: 250
- Protein: 28g
- Carbohydrates: 12g
- Sugars: 7g
- Dietary Fiber: 3g
- Fat: 11g
- Sodium: 75mg
- Potassium: 420mg
- Phosphorus: 220mg

2. Tuna Salad Wrap with Cucumber

👥 2 | ⏱ 10 min | 🍽 0 min

Ingredients:

- 1 can low-sodium tuna, drained
- 2 tbsp plain Greek yogurt
- 1 tbsp lemon juice
- 1/4 cup diced cucumber
- 1/4 cup diced celery
- 2 low-sodium whole grain tortillas

- Fresh dill (optional)

Instructions:

1. In a bowl, combine tuna, Greek yogurt, lemon juice, cucumber, and celery. Mix well.
2. Spoon tuna mixture onto the center of each tortilla.
3. Sprinkle with fresh dill if using.
4. Roll up the tortillas and slice in half. Serve immediately.

Nutritional Information (per serving):

- Calories: 210
- Protein: 24g
- Carbohydrates: 20g
- Sugars: 3g
- Dietary Fiber: 4g
- Fat: 6g
- Sodium: 150mg
- Potassium: 290mg
- Phosphorus: 200mg

3. Low-Sodium Lentil Soup

👥 4 | ⏱ 15 min | 🍲 30 min

Ingredients:

- 1 cup dried lentils, rinsed
- 1 small onion, diced
- 2 cloves garlic, minced
- 1 carrot, diced
- 1 celery stalk, diced
- 6 cups low-sodium vegetable broth
- 1 tsp ground cumin
- 1/2 tsp ground coriander
- 2 tbsp olive oil
- Fresh parsley, chopped (for garnish)

Instructions:

1. In a large pot, heat olive oil over medium heat. Add onion, garlic, carrot, and celery. Sauté until softened.
2. Stir in lentils, cumin, and coriander.
3. Add vegetable broth and bring to a boil.
4. Reduce heat and simmer for 25-30 minutes, or until lentils are tender.
5. Ladle soup into bowls and garnish with fresh parsley. Serve warm.

Nutritional Information (per serving):

- Calories: 180
- Protein: 10g
- Carbohydrates: 25g
- Sugars: 4g
- Dietary Fiber: 8g
- Fat: 6g
- Sodium: 75mg
- Potassium: 350mg
- Phosphorus: 180mg

4. Veggie and Hummus Pita Pocket

👥 2 | ⏱ 10 min | 🍲 0 min

Ingredients:

- 2 whole grain pita pockets
- 1/2 cup hummus (low-sodium)
- 1/4 cup sliced cucumbers
- 1/4 cup shredded carrots
- 1/4 cup sliced bell peppers
- 1/4 cup spinach leaves
- 1 tbsp olive oil
- Fresh lemon juice (optional)

Instructions:

1. Carefully open each pita pocket.
2. Spread hummus inside each pita.
3. Fill with sliced cucumbers, shredded carrots, bell peppers, and spinach leaves.
4. Drizzle with olive oil and fresh lemon juice if desired. Serve immediately.

Nutritional Information (per serving):

- Calories: 220
- Protein: 7g
- Carbohydrates: 30g
- Sugars: 5g
- Dietary Fiber: 8g
- Fat: 9g
- Sodium: 120mg
- Potassium: 320mg
- Phosphorus: 160mg

5. Turkey and Avocado Sandwich

👥 1 | ⏱ 5 min | 🍲 0 min

Ingredients:

- 2 slices low-sodium whole grain bread
- 2 oz sliced turkey breast (low-sodium)
- 1/4 avocado, sliced
- 1 leaf lettuce
- 2 slices tomato

1 tsp Dijon mustard (optional)

Instructions:

1. Spread Dijon mustard on one slice of bread if using.
2. Layer turkey, avocado slices, lettuce, and tomato on the bread.
3. Top with the second slice of bread. Serve immediately.

Nutritional Information (per serving):

- Calories: 230
- Protein: 14g
- Carbohydrates: 24g
- Sugars: 3g
- Dietary Fiber: 6g
- Fat: 10g
- Sodium: 130mg
- Potassium: 350mg
- Phosphorus: 180mg

6. Quinoa and Black Bean Salad

👥 2 | ⏱ 10 min | 🍳 15 min

Ingredients:

- 1/2 cup cooked quinoa
- 1/2 cup black beans (no salt added), rinsed
- 1/4 cup corn kernels
- 1/4 cup diced red bell pepper
- 1/4 cup diced avocado
- 2 tbsp chopped cilantro
- 1 tbsp olive oil
- 1 tbsp lime juice
- 1/4 tsp ground cumin

Instructions:

1. In a large bowl, combine quinoa, black beans, corn, bell pepper, and avocado.
2. In a small bowl, whisk together olive oil, lime juice, and cumin.
3. Pour dressing over the salad and toss gently to combine.

4. Garnish with chopped cilantro and serve.

Nutritional Information (per serving):

- Calories: 250
- Protein: 7g
- Carbohydrates: 35g
- Sugars: 2g
- Dietary Fiber: 9g
- Fat: 10g
- Sodium: 45mg
- Potassium: 450mg
- Phosphorus: 190mg

7. Chicken and Spinach Wrap

👥 2 | ⏱ 10 min | 🍳 0 min

Ingredients:

- 2 low-sodium whole grain tortillas
- 1 cup cooked chicken breast, shredded
- 1/2 cup fresh spinach leaves
- 1/4 cup grated carrots
- 1/4 avocado, sliced
- 1 tbsp plain Greek yogurt
- Fresh lemon juice (optional)

Instructions:

1. Lay out tortillas and spread Greek yogurt evenly.
2. Layer spinach leaves, shredded chicken, grated carrots, and avocado slices.
3. Drizzle with fresh lemon juice if desired.
4. Roll up the tortillas, slice in half, and serve.

Nutritional Information (per serving):

- Calories: 290
- Protein: 25g
- Carbohydrates: 20g
- Sugars: 2g
- Dietary Fiber: 5g
- Fat: 13g
- Sodium: 90mg
- Potassium: 420mg
- Phosphorus: 250mg

8. Mediterranean Couscous Salad

👥 2 | ⏱ 10 min | 🍳 10 min

Ingredients:

Chapter 5: Lunch Recipes

- 1/2 cup cooked whole wheat couscous
- 1/4 cup cherry tomatoes, halved
- 1/4 cup diced cucumber
- 1/4 cup crumbled feta cheese (optional, reduce for lower sodium)
- 2 tbsp chopped kalamata olives (optional)
- 2 tbsp olive oil
- 1 tbsp red wine vinegar
- Fresh basil leaves for garnish

Instructions:

1. In a large bowl, combine couscous, cherry tomatoes, cucumber, feta cheese, and olives.
2. In a small bowl, whisk together olive oil and red wine vinegar.
3. Pour dressing over the salad and toss gently to combine.
4. Garnish with fresh basil leaves and serve.

Nutritional Information (per serving):

- Calories: 240
- Protein: 6g
- Carbohydrates: 28g
- Sugars: 4g
- Dietary Fiber: 4g
- Fat: 12g
- Sodium: 200mg
- Potassium: 300mg
- Phosphorus: 160mg

9. Shrimp and Avocado Salad

👥 2 | ⏱ 10 min | 🍽 5 min

Ingredients:

- 1/2 lb shrimp, peeled and deveined
- 1/4 avocado, diced
- 1/2 cup cherry tomatoes, halved
- 1/4 cup diced cucumber
- 1/4 cup diced red onion
- 2 tbsp olive oil
- 1 tbsp fresh lemon juice
- Fresh cilantro leaves for garnish

Instructions:

1. In a medium pan, sauté shrimp in 1 tbsp olive oil until pink and fully cooked, about 3-4 minutes.
2. In a large bowl, combine avocado, cherry tomatoes, cucumber, and red onion.
3. Add cooked shrimp to the bowl.
4. Drizzle with remaining olive oil and lemon juice. Toss gently to combine.
5. Garnish with cilantro leaves and serve.

Nutritional Information (per serving):

- Calories: 250
- Protein: 20g
- Carbohydrates: 8g
- Sugars: 3g
- Dietary Fiber: 4g
- Fat: 15g
- Sodium: 150mg
- Potassium: 370mg
- Phosphorus: 220mg

10. Pasta Salad with Roasted Vegetables

👥 2 | ⏱ 15 min | 🍽 20 min

Ingredients:

- 1 cup whole wheat pasta
- 1/2 cup zucchini, sliced
- 1/2 cup cherry tomatoes
- 1/4 cup diced red onion
- 1/4 cup diced bell pepper
- 2 tbsp olive oil
- 1 tbsp balsamic vinegar
- 1/4 tsp dried oregano
- Fresh basil leaves for garnish

Instructions:

1. Cook pasta according to package instructions. Drain and set aside.
2. Preheat oven to 400°F (200°C). On a baking sheet, toss zucchini, cherry tomatoes, red onion, and bell pepper with 1 tbsp olive oil.
3. Roast vegetables for 15-20 minutes, until tender and slightly charred.
4. In a large bowl, combine cooked pasta with roasted vegetables.
5. In a small bowl, whisk together remaining olive oil, balsamic vinegar, and oregano.
6. Pour dressing over pasta salad, toss gently, and garnish with fresh basil leaves. Serve warm or chilled.

Nutritional Information (per serving):

- Calories: 280
- Protein: 8g
- Carbohydrates: 42g
- Sugars: 6g
- Dietary Fiber: 7g
- Fat: 10g
- Sodium: 60mg
- Potassium: 450mg
- Phosphorus: 190mg

11. Chicken Caesar Salad (Lightened Up)

👥 2 | ⏱ 10 min | 🍲 0 min

Ingredients:

- 2 cups chopped romaine lettuce
- 1 cup cooked chicken breast, diced
- 1/4 cup shaved Parmesan cheese (optional)
- 1/4 cup croutons (low-sodium)
- 2 tbsp light Caesar dressing
- Fresh lemon wedges (for serving)

Instructions:

1. In a large bowl, combine romaine lettuce, diced chicken, Parmesan cheese, and croutons.
2. Drizzle with light Caesar dressing and toss gently to coat.
3. Serve with lemon wedges on the side.

Nutritional Information (per serving):

- Calories: 260
- Protein: 25g
- Carbohydrates: 10g
- Sugars: 2g
- Dietary Fiber: 3g
- Fat: 12g
- Sodium: 180mg
- Potassium: 380mg
- Phosphorus: 220mg

12. Egg Salad Lettuce Wraps

👥 2 | ⏱ 10 min | 🍲 0 min

Ingredients:

- 4 hard-boiled eggs, chopped
- 2 tbsp plain Greek yogurt
- 1 tbsp Dijon mustard
- 1 tbsp chopped chives
- 4 large lettuce leaves
- Fresh dill for garnish (optional)

Instructions:

1. In a bowl, mix chopped eggs with Greek yogurt, Dijon mustard, and chives.
2. Spoon egg salad into the center of each lettuce leaf.
3. Garnish with fresh dill if desired. Serve immediately.

Nutritional Information (per serving):

- Calories: 220
- Protein: 15g
- Carbohydrates: 3g
- Sugars: 1g
- Dietary Fiber: 1g
- Fat: 18g
- Sodium: 160mg
- Potassium: 140mg
- Phosphorus: 230mg

13. Spaghetti Squash with Pesto

👥 2 | ⏱ 10 min | 🍲 40 min

Ingredients:

- 1 medium spaghetti squash
- 1/4 cup basil pesto (low-sodium)
- 2 tbsp grated Parmesan cheese (optional)
- 1 tbsp olive oil
- Fresh basil leaves for garnish

Instructions:

1. Preheat oven to 400°F (200°C). Cut spaghetti squash in half and remove seeds.
2. Drizzle with olive oil and place cut-side down on a baking sheet. Roast for 35-40 minutes, until tender.
3. Use a fork to scrape out the squash into strands.
4. In a large bowl, toss squash with pesto and Parmesan cheese.
5. Garnish with fresh basil leaves and serve warm.

Nutritional Information (per serving):

- Calories: 180
- Protein: 5g
- Carbohydrates: 16g

- Sugars: 4g
- Dietary Fiber: 4g
- Fat: 12g
- Sodium: 150mg
- Potassium: 420mg
- Phosphorus: 120mg

14. BBQ Tofu Salad

👥 2 | ⏱ 10 min | 🍲 15 min

Ingredients:

- 1 block firm tofu, pressed and cubed
- 1/4 cup BBQ sauce (low-sodium)
- 4 cups mixed salad greens
- 1/4 cup shredded carrots
- 1/4 cup sliced red onion
- 1/4 cup diced cucumber
- 2 tbsp olive oil
- Fresh cilantro for garnish

Instructions:

1. In a large pan, heat olive oil over medium heat. Add cubed tofu and cook until golden on all sides.
2. Add BBQ sauce to the pan and toss tofu to coat evenly.
3. In a large bowl, combine salad greens, shredded carrots, red onion, and cucumber.
4. Top with BBQ tofu and garnish with fresh cilantro. Serve immediately.

Nutritional Information (per serving):

- Calories: 240
- Protein: 15g
- Carbohydrates: 15g
- Sugars: 7g
- Dietary Fiber: 5g
- Fat: 13g
- Sodium: 180mg
- Potassium: 320mg
- Phosphorus: 190mg

15. Turkey and Sweet Potato Bowl

👥 2 | ⏱ 15 min | 🍲 25 min

Ingredients:

- 1 large sweet potato, peeled and diced
- 1 cup cooked ground turkey (low-sodium)
- 1/2 cup cooked quinoa
- 1/4 cup diced avocado
- 2 tbsp olive oil
- 1 tbsp lime juice
- Fresh cilantro for garnish

Instructions:

1. Preheat oven to 400°F (200°C). Toss diced sweet potato with 1 tbsp olive oil and roast for 20-25 minutes, until tender.
2. In a large bowl, combine cooked ground turkey, roasted sweet potato, and cooked quinoa.
3. Drizzle with remaining olive oil and lime juice.
4. Top with diced avocado and garnish with fresh cilantro. Serve warm.

Nutritional Information (per serving):

- Calories: 320
- Protein: 20g
- Carbohydrates: 35g
- Sugars: 7g
- Dietary Fiber: 8g
- Fat: 14g
- Sodium: 90mg
- Potassium: 550mg
- Phosphorus: 240m

16. Spiced Chickpea Salad Wrap

👥 2 | ⏱ 10 min | 🍲 0 min

Ingredients:

- 1 cup canned chickpeas, rinsed and drained
- 1/4 cup diced cucumber
- 1/4 cup diced red bell pepper
- 1 tbsp lemon juice
- 1/2 tsp ground cumin
- 1/4 tsp paprika
- 2 low-sodium whole grain tortillas

Instructions:

1. In a bowl, mix chickpeas, cucumber, bell pepper, lemon juice, cumin, and paprika.
2. Spoon the chickpea mixture onto the tortillas.
3. Wrap tightly and serve.

Nutritional Information (per serving):

- Calories: 220

- Protein: 7g
- Carbohydrates: 35g
- Sugars: 3g
- Dietary Fiber: 8g
- Fat: 5g
- Sodium: 40mg
- Potassium: 250mg
- Phosphorus: 80mg

17. Lentil and Vegetable Soup

👥 4 | ⏱ 15 min | 🍲 30 min

Ingredients:

- 1 cup dry lentils, rinsed
- 1/2 cup diced carrots
- 1/2 cup diced celery
- 1/2 cup diced tomatoes
- 1 clove garlic, minced
- 4 cups low-sodium vegetable broth
- 1 tbsp olive oil

Instructions:

1. Heat olive oil in a pot over medium heat.
2. Sauté garlic, carrots, and celery until tender.
3. Add lentils, tomatoes, and broth. Bring to a boil.
4. Reduce heat and simmer for 30 minutes, until lentils are tender.

Nutritional Information (per serving):

- Calories: 180
- Protein: 9g
- Carbohydrates: 30g
- Sugars: 4g
- Dietary Fiber: 8g
- Fat: 3g
- Sodium: 100mg
- Potassium: 350mg
- Phosphorus: 120mg

18. Quinoa and Avocado Salad

👥 2 | ⏱ 10 min | 🍲 0 min

Ingredients:

- 1 cup cooked quinoa
- 1/2 avocado, diced
- 1/4 cup cherry tomatoes, halved
- 1 tbsp lemon juice
- 1 tbsp olive oil
- 1/4 tsp black pepper

Instructions:

1. In a bowl, combine quinoa, avocado, cherry tomatoes, lemon juice, and olive oil.
2. Toss gently and season with black pepper. Serve immediately.

Nutritional Information (per serving):

- Calories: 220
- Protein: 6g
- Carbohydrates: 26g
- Sugars: 3g
- Dietary Fiber: 5g
- Fat: 10g
- Sodium: 15mg
- Potassium: 300mg
- Phosphorus: 90mg

19. Baked Turkey and Veggie Roll-Ups

👥 2 | ⏱ 10 min | 🍲 15 min

Ingredients:

- 4 slices turkey breast, low-sodium
- 1/2 cup spinach leaves
- 1/2 cup shredded carrots
- 2 tbsp low-fat cream cheese

Instructions:

1. Preheat oven to 350°F (175°C).
2. Spread cream cheese on turkey slices.
3. Place spinach and carrots on each slice and roll up.
4. Bake for 15 minutes, until heated through.

Nutritional Information (per serving):

- Calories: 150
- Protein: 14g
- Carbohydrates: 5g
- Sugars: 2g
- Dietary Fiber: 1g
- Fat: 7g
- Sodium: 180mg
- Potassium: 180mg
- Phosphorus: 100mg

Chapter 5: Lunch Recipes

20. Zucchini Noodles with Pesto
👥 2 | ⏱ 10 min | 🍲 5 min

Ingredients:
- 2 medium zucchinis, spiralized
- 2 tbsp basil pesto (low-sodium)
- 1 tbsp olive oil

Instructions:
1. Heat olive oil in a skillet over medium heat.
2. Add zucchini noodles and sauté for 3-5 minutes until tender.
3. Toss with pesto and serve warm.

Nutritional Information (per serving):
- Calories: 140
- Protein: 2g
- Carbohydrates: 8g
- Sugars: 4g
- Dietary Fiber: 2g
- Fat: 12g
- Sodium: 60mg
- Potassium: 220mg
- Phosphorus: 40mg

21. Lemon Chicken and Rice Salad
👥 2 | ⏱ 15 min | 🍲 20 min

Ingredients:
- 1/2 cup cooked brown rice
- 1/2 cup diced cooked chicken breast
- 1/4 cup diced cucumber
- 1 tbsp lemon juice
- 1 tbsp olive oil
- 1/4 tsp dried oregano

Instructions:
1. In a large bowl, combine rice, chicken, and cucumber.
2. Drizzle with lemon juice and olive oil. Sprinkle with oregano.
3. Toss gently and serve.

Nutritional Information (per serving):
- Calories: 230
- Protein: 15g
- Carbohydrates: 25g
- Sugars: 1g
- Dietary Fiber: 3g
- Fat: 8g
- Sodium: 45mg
- Potassium: 200mg
- Phosphorus: 150mg

22. Spinach and Feta Stuffed Pita
👥 2 | ⏱ 10 min | 🍲 0 min

Ingredients:
- 2 whole wheat pita pockets
- 1/2 cup fresh spinach leaves
- 1/4 cup crumbled feta cheese (low-sodium)
- 1/4 cup diced tomatoes

Instructions:
1. Stuff each pita pocket with spinach, feta cheese, and tomatoes.
2. Serve immediately.

Nutritional Information (per serving):
- Calories: 180
- Protein: 6g
- Carbohydrates: 24g
- Sugars: 2g
- Dietary Fiber: 4g
- Fat: 7g
- Sodium: 140mg
- Potassium: 150mg
- Phosphorus: 90mg

23. Veggie Quinoa Pilaf
👥 4 | ⏱ 15 min | 🍲 20 min

Ingredients:
- 1 cup quinoa, rinsed
- 1/2 cup diced zucchini
- 1/2 cup diced carrots
- 1/4 cup diced onion
- 1 tbsp olive oil
- 2 cups low-sodium vegetable broth

Instructions:
1. Heat olive oil in a pot over medium heat.
2. Sauté onion, zucchini, and carrots until tender.
3. Add quinoa and broth, bring to a boil.
4. Reduce heat, cover, and simmer for 20 minutes.

Nutritional Information (per serving):

- Calories: 150
- Protein: 5g
- Carbohydrates: 25g
- Sugars: 3g
- Dietary Fiber: 4g
- Fat: 4g
- Sodium: 60mg
- Potassium: 180mg
- Phosphorus: 100mg

24. Mediterranean Chickpea Salad
👥 4 | ⏱ 10 min | 🍲 0 min

Ingredients:
- 1 cup canned chickpeas, rinsed and drained
- 1/2 cup cherry tomatoes, halved
- 1/4 cup diced cucumber
- 1/4 cup black olives, sliced (optional)
- 1 tbsp olive oil
- 1 tbsp lemon juice

Instructions:
1. In a large bowl, combine chickpeas, tomatoes, cucumber, and olives.
2. Drizzle with olive oil and lemon juice. Toss gently.
3. Serve chilled.

Nutritional Information (per serving):
- Calories: 110
- Protein: 4g
- Carbohydrates: 16g
- Sugars: 2g
- Dietary Fiber: 4g
- Fat: 5g
- Sodium: 50mg
- Potassium: 150mg
- Phosphorus: 80mg

25. Sweet Potato and Black Bean Tacos
👥 2 | ⏱ 15 min | 🍲 15 min

Ingredients:
- 1 medium sweet potato, peeled and cubed
- 1/2 cup canned black beans, rinsed
- 1/4 tsp ground cumin
- 1/4 tsp chili powder
- 4 corn tortillas (low-sodium)
- 1 tbsp olive oil

Instructions:
1. Preheat oven to 375°F (190°C).
2. Toss sweet potato cubes with olive oil, cumin, and chili powder.
3. Bake for 15 minutes or until tender.
4. Fill tortillas with sweet potatoes and black beans.

Nutritional Information (per serving):
- Calories: 200
- Protein: 6g
- Carbohydrates: 35g
- Sugars: 5g
- Dietary Fiber: 7g
- Fat: 5g
- Sodium: 80mg
- Potassium: 300mg
- Phosphorus: 90mg

26. Turkey Avocado Lettuce Wraps
👥 2 | ⏱ 10 min | 🍲 0 min

Ingredients:
- 4 large lettuce leaves (e.g., romaine or butter lettuce)
- 4 slices low-sodium turkey breast
- 1/2 avocado, sliced
- 1/4 cup shredded carrots
- 1 tbsp hummus (low-sodium)

Instructions:
1. Lay out lettuce leaves on a flat surface.
2. Spread a thin layer of hummus on each leaf.
3. Top with turkey slices, avocado, and shredded carrots.
4. Roll each leaf tightly to form a wrap. Serve immediately.

Nutritional Information (per serving):
- Calories: 150
- Protein: 10g
- Carbohydrates: 8g
- Sugars: 2g
- Dietary Fiber: 4g
- Fat: 8g

Chapter 5: Lunch Recipes

- Sodium: 180mg
- Potassium: 240mg
- Phosphorus: 100mg

27. Grilled Vegetable Panini

👥 2 | ⏱ 15 min | 🍲 10 min

Ingredients:

- 4 slices low-sodium whole grain bread
- 1/2 cup zucchini, sliced
- 1/2 cup red bell pepper, sliced
- 1/2 cup eggplant, sliced
- 2 tbsp low-fat cream cheese
- 1 tbsp olive oil

Instructions:

1. Preheat a grill or skillet over medium heat.
2. Brush vegetables with olive oil and grill until tender, about 5 minutes per side.
3. Spread cream cheese on two slices of bread.
4. Layer grilled vegetables between bread slices to form sandwiches.
5. Grill sandwiches for 3-4 minutes on each side or until golden brown. Serve warm.

Nutritional Information (per serving):

- Calories: 230
- Protein: 8g
- Carbohydrates: 32g
- Sugars: 4g
- Dietary Fiber: 6g
- Fat: 8g
- Sodium: 140mg
- Potassium: 280mg
- Phosphorus: 100mg

28. Shrimp and Cucumber Salad

👥 2 | ⏱ 10 min | 🍲 0 min

Ingredients:

- 8 large shrimp, cooked and chilled
- 1 cup cucumber, diced
- 1/4 cup red onion, finely chopped
- 2 tbsp lemon juice
- 1 tbsp fresh dill, chopped

Instructions:

1. In a large bowl, combine shrimp, cucumber, and red onion.
2. Drizzle with lemon juice and sprinkle with dill. Toss gently and serve chilled.

Nutritional Information (per serving):

- Calories: 110
- Protein: 12g
- Carbohydrates: 6g
- Sugars: 2g
- Dietary Fiber: 1g
- Fat: 4g
- Sodium: 150mg
- Potassium: 200mg
- Phosphorus: 120mg

29. Lentil and Quinoa Stuffed Peppers

👥 2 | ⏱ 15 min | 🍲 30 min

Ingredients:

- 2 large bell peppers, halved and seeded
- 1/2 cup cooked lentils
- 1/2 cup cooked quinoa
- 1/4 cup diced tomatoes
- 1/4 tsp cumin
- 1 tbsp olive oil

Instructions:

1. Preheat oven to 375°F (190°C).
2. In a bowl, mix lentils, quinoa, tomatoes, cumin, and olive oil.
3. Stuff each bell pepper half with the mixture and place in a baking dish.
4. Bake for 30 minutes, or until peppers are tender. Serve warm.

Nutritional Information (per serving):

- Calories: 200
- Protein: 8g
- Carbohydrates: 30g
- Sugars: 6g
- Dietary Fiber: 7g
- Fat: 5g
- Sodium: 40mg
- Potassium: 350mg
- Phosphorus: 110mg

30. Greek Yogurt Chicken Salad

👥 2 | ⏱ 10 min | 🍲 0 min

Ingredients:

- 1 cup cooked chicken breast, diced
- 1/2 cup plain Greek yogurt (low-sodium)
- 1/4 cup celery, chopped
- 1/4 cup apple, diced
- 1 tbsp lemon juice
- 1/2 tsp dried dill

Instructions:

1. In a bowl, combine chicken, Greek yogurt, celery, apple, lemon juice, and dill.
2. Mix well and serve chilled, on its own or with a side of lettuce leaves.

Nutritional Information (per serving):

- Calories: 180
- Protein: 20g
- Carbohydrates: 10g
- Sugars: 5g
- Dietary Fiber: 1g
- Fat: 6g
- Sodium: 60mg
- Potassium: 210mg
- Phosphorus: 150mg

Lunch Tips and Tricks

Finding time to prepare a healthy, kidney-friendly lunch doesn't have to be stressful. Here are some tips to make lunchtime easier:

- **Batch Cooking**: Prepare larger portions of your favorite lunch recipes, so you have leftovers ready for the next day. Soups, salads, and wraps are perfect for this.
- **Pack Ahead**: If you're heading to work or running errands, pack your lunch the night before. This way, you won't be tempted to grab something less healthy on the go.
- **Mix and Match**: Combine different recipes to create a variety of lunches throughout the week. This keeps your meals exciting and ensures you're getting a balanced diet.
- **Hydration Reminder**: Always pair your lunch with a hydrating drink like water, herbal tea, or a low-sodium broth.

By incorporating these lunch recipes into your routine, you'll enjoy flavorful, satisfying meals that support your kidney health. Lunchtime will become a moment of nourishment and pleasure, helping you stay on track with your renal diet goals.

Chapter 6: Dinner Recipes

End Your Day Right: Nourishing Dinner Ideas

Dinner is often the meal where you unwind and reflect on the day. It's your opportunity to enjoy a hearty, satisfying meal that wraps up your day on a high note. When following a renal diet, it's essential to make dinner both nutritious and delicious, ensuring you end the day with food that supports your kidney health without sacrificing flavor.

This chapter is packed with a variety of dinner recipes that are perfect for a quiet night at home or sharing with family and friends. From comforting classics to creative new dishes, these meals are designed to be low in sodium, potassium, and phosphorus, making them ideal for a kidney-friendly diet.

Let's dive into these dinner recipes that will help you wind down your day with satisfaction and nourishment.

30 Kidney-Friendly Dinner Recipes

1. Baked Lemon Herb Chicken

4 | 10 min | 30 min

Ingredients:

- 4 boneless, skinless chicken breasts
- 2 tbsp olive oil
- 1 lemon, sliced
- 2 cloves garlic, minced
- 1 tsp dried oregano
- 1 tsp dried thyme
- Fresh parsley for garnish

Instructions:

1. Preheat oven to 375°F (190°C).
2. Place chicken breasts in a baking dish. Drizzle with olive oil and top with lemon slices.
3. Sprinkle garlic, oregano, and thyme over the chicken.
4. Bake for 25-30 minutes, until the chicken is fully cooked.
5. Garnish with fresh parsley and serve.

Nutritional Information (per serving):

- Calories: 220
- Protein: 28g
- Carbohydrates: 2g
- Sugars: 0g
- Dietary Fiber: 1g
- Fat: 11g
- Sodium: 60mg
- Potassium: 350mg
- Phosphorus: 220mg

2. Grilled Salmon with Dill Sauce

2 | 10 min | 15 min

Ingredients:

- 2 salmon fillets
- 1 tbsp olive oil
- 1 tbsp fresh lemon juice
- 1/4 cup plain Greek yogurt
- 1 tbsp fresh dill, chopped
- 1/2 tsp lemon zest
- Black pepper to taste

Instructions:

1. Preheat grill to medium-high heat.
2. Brush salmon fillets with olive oil and lemon juice. Season with black pepper.
3. Grill salmon for 4-5 minutes per side, until cooked through.
4. In a small bowl, mix Greek yogurt, dill, and lemon zest to make the dill sauce.
5. Serve the salmon topped with the dill sauce.

Nutritional Information (per serving):

- Calories: 290
- Protein: 26g

- Carbohydrates: 3g
- Sugars: 1g
- Dietary Fiber: 0g
- Fat: 19g
- Sodium: 70mg
- Potassium: 420mg
- Phosphorus: 260mg

3. Grilled Salmon with Avocado Salsa

👥 2 | ⏱ 10 min | 🍽 10 min

Ingredients:

- 2 salmon fillets
- 1 ripe avocado, diced
- 1/2 cup cherry tomatoes, halved
- 1/4 red onion, finely chopped
- 1 tbsp fresh cilantro, chopped
- 1 tbsp lime juice
- 1 tsp olive oil
- Salt and pepper to taste

Instructions:

6. Preheat grill to medium-high heat.
1. Drizzle salmon fillets with olive oil and season with salt and pepper.
2. Grill salmon for 4-5 minutes per side, until cooked through and flakey.
3. In a bowl, combine diced avocado, cherry tomatoes, red onion, cilantro, and lime juice. Stir gently.
4. Serve the grilled salmon topped with the avocado salsa.

Nutritional Information (per serving):

- Calories: 350
- Protein: 30g
- Carbohydrates: 15g
- Sugars: 5g
- Dietary Fiber: 7g
- Fat: 22g
- Sodium: 120mg
- Potassium: 850mg
- Phosphorus: 350mg

4. Vegetarian Stir-Fry with Tofu

👥 2 | ⏱ 15 min | 🍽 20 min

Ingredients:

- 1 block firm tofu, pressed and cubed
- 1 cup broccoli florets
- 1 red bell pepper, sliced
- 1 zucchini, sliced
- 2 tbsp low-sodium soy sauce
- 1 tbsp sesame oil
- 1 tbsp fresh ginger, minced
- 1 clove garlic, minced
- 1 tbsp sesame seeds (optional)

Instructions:

1. Heat sesame oil in a large pan or wok over medium heat. Add tofu and cook until golden brown on all sides.
2. Remove tofu from the pan and set aside.
3. In the same pan, add garlic and ginger, and sauté for 1 minute.
4. Add broccoli, bell pepper, and zucchini, and stir-fry for 5-7 minutes until tender.
5. Return tofu to the pan and stir in soy sauce. Cook for an additional 2 minutes.
6. Garnish with sesame seeds if desired and serve.

Nutritional Information (per serving):

- Calories: 240
- Protein: 14g
- Carbohydrates: 16g
- Sugars: 5g
- Dietary Fiber: 4g
- Fat: 14g
- Sodium: 120mg
- Potassium: 420mg
- Phosphorus: 170mg

5. Baked Cod with Lemon and Garlic

👥 4 | ⏱ 10 min | 🍽 20 min

Ingredients:

- 4 cod fillets
- 2 tbsp olive oil
- 2 cloves garlic, minced
- 1 lemon, juiced
- 1 tsp dried parsley
- Black pepper to taste

Instructions:

Chapter 6: Dinner Recipes

1. Preheat oven to 375°F (190°C).
2. Place cod fillets in a baking dish. Drizzle with olive oil and lemon juice.
3. Sprinkle garlic, parsley, and black pepper over the fillets.
4. Bake for 18-20 minutes, until the fish flakes easily with a fork.

Nutritional Information (per serving):

- Calories: 200
- Protein: 28g
- Carbohydrates: 1g
- Sugars: 0g
- Dietary Fiber: 0g
- Fat: 9g
- Sodium: 60mg
- Potassium: 490mg
- Phosphorus: 250mg

6. Turkey Meatballs with Zucchini Noodles

👥 4 | ⏱ 20 min | 🍲 30 min

Ingredients:

- 1 lb ground turkey
- 1/2 cup breadcrumbs (low-sodium)
- 1 egg white
- 1/4 cup grated Parmesan cheese (optional)
- 2 cloves garlic, minced
- 1 tsp dried basil
- 1 tsp dried oregano
- 4 medium zucchinis, spiralized
- 2 tbsp olive oil

Instructions:

1. Preheat oven to 375°F (190°C).
2. In a large bowl, combine ground turkey, breadcrumbs, egg white, Parmesan cheese, garlic, basil, and oregano. Mix well.
3. Form mixture into small meatballs and place on a baking sheet.
4. Bake for 25-30 minutes, until cooked through.
5. In a large pan, heat olive oil over medium heat. Add spiralized zucchini and sauté for 3-4 minutes until tender.
6. Serve meatballs over zucchini noodles.

Nutritional Information (per serving):

- Calories: 290
- Protein: 28g
- Carbohydrates: 10g
- Sugars: 4g
- Dietary Fiber: 3g
- Fat: 14g
- Sodium: 90mg
- Potassium: 450mg
- Phosphorus: 210mg

7. Quinoa-Stuffed Portobello Mushrooms

👥 4 | ⏱ 15 min | 🍲 25 min

Ingredients:

- 4 large portobello mushrooms, stems removed
- 1 cup cooked quinoa
- 1/2 cup diced tomatoes
- 1/4 cup chopped spinach
- 1/4 cup shredded mozzarella cheese (optional)
- 2 tbsp olive oil
- 1 clove garlic, minced
- 1 tsp dried basil

Instructions:

1. Preheat oven to 375°F (190°C).
2. In a large bowl, combine quinoa, diced tomatoes, spinach, garlic, basil, and olive oil. Mix well.
3. Stuff each mushroom cap with the quinoa mixture and place on a baking sheet.
4. Top with shredded mozzarella cheese if desired.
5. Bake for 20-25 minutes, until the mushrooms are tender and the cheese is melted.

Nutritional Information (per serving):

- Calories: 210
- Protein: 9g
- Carbohydrates: 20g
- Sugars: 4g
- Dietary Fiber: 5g
- Fat: 10g
- Sodium: 80mg
- Potassium: 550mg
- Phosphorus: 180mg

8. Garlic Shrimp with Asparagus
👥 2 | ⏱ 10 min | 🍽 10 min

Ingredients:
- 1/2 lb shrimp, peeled and deveined
- 1 bunch asparagus, trimmed and cut into 2-inch pieces
- 2 cloves garlic, minced
- 2 tbsp olive oil
- 1 tbsp fresh lemon juice
- Black pepper to taste

Instructions:
1. In a large pan, heat olive oil over medium heat. Add garlic and sauté for 1 minute.
2. Add shrimp and asparagus to the pan and cook for 4-5 minutes, until the shrimp are pink and the asparagus is tender.
3. Drizzle with lemon juice and season with black pepper. Serve immediately.

Nutritional Information (per serving):
- Calories: 220
- Protein: 24g
- Carbohydrates: 6g
- Sugars: 2g
- Dietary Fiber: 3g
- Fat: 11g
- Sodium: 140mg
- Potassium: 380mg
- Phosphorus: 210mg

9. Balsamic-Glazed Chicken with Brussels Sprouts
👥 2 | ⏱ 15 min | 🍽 25 min

Ingredients:
- 2 boneless, skinless chicken breasts
- 1/2 lb Brussels sprouts, halved
- 2 tbsp balsamic vinegar
- 1 tbsp olive oil
- 1 tbsp honey
- 2 cloves garlic, minced
- Black pepper to taste

Instructions:
1. Preheat oven to 400°F (200°C).
2. In a small bowl, whisk together balsamic vinegar, honey, garlic, and olive oil.
3. Place chicken breasts and Brussels sprouts in a baking dish. Drizzle with balsamic mixture and toss to coat.
4. Bake for 20-25 minutes, until the chicken is cooked through and the Brussels sprouts are tender.

Nutritional Information (per serving):
- Calories: 280
- Protein: 28g
- Carbohydrates: 18g
- Sugars: 10g
- Dietary Fiber: 5g
- Fat: 10g
- Sodium: 100mg
- Potassium: 450mg
- Phosphorus: 220mg

10. Turkey Chili
👥 4 | ⏱ 15 min | 🍽 40 min

Ingredients:
- 1 lb ground turkey
- 1 can low-sodium kidney beans, rinsed
- 1 can low-sodium diced tomatoes
- 1 small onion, diced
- 2 cloves garlic, minced
- 1 tbsp chili powder
- 1 tsp ground cumin
- 1 tsp paprika
- 2 tbsp olive oil

Instructions:
1. In a large pot, heat olive oil over medium heat. Add onion and garlic, and sauté until softened.
2. Add ground turkey and cook until browned.
3. Stir in kidney beans, diced tomatoes, chili powder, cumin, and paprika.
4. Bring to a boil, then reduce heat and simmer for 30-35 minutes.
5. Serve warm.

Nutritional Information (per serving):
- Calories: 290
- Protein: 28g
- Carbohydrates: 24g

- Sugars: 5g
- Dietary Fiber: 8g
- Fat: 10g
- Sodium: 120mg
- Potassium: 420mg
- Phosphorus: 240mg

11. Baked Eggplant Parmesan

👥 4 | ⏱ 20 min | 🍲 40 min

Ingredients:

- 1 large eggplant, sliced into rounds
- 1/2 cup breadcrumbs (low-sodium)
- 1/4 cup grated Parmesan cheese
- 1 cup low-sodium tomato sauce
- 1 cup shredded mozzarella cheese (optional)
- 2 tbsp olive oil
- 1 tsp dried oregano
- Fresh basil leaves for garnish

Instructions:

1. Preheat oven to 375°F (190°C).
2. In a bowl, mix breadcrumbs with Parmesan cheese and oregano.
3. Brush eggplant slices with olive oil and coat with breadcrumb mixture.
4. Place eggplant slices on a baking sheet and bake for 20-25 minutes until golden brown.
5. In a baking dish, layer eggplant slices with tomato sauce and mozzarella cheese.
6. Bake for an additional 15-20 minutes until the cheese is melted and bubbly.
7. Garnish with fresh basil leaves and serve.

Nutritional Information (per serving):

- Calories: 280
- Protein: 10g
- Carbohydrates: 30g
- Sugars: 7g
- Dietary Fiber: 7g
- Fat: 13g
- Sodium: 150mg
- Potassium: 600mg
- Phosphorus: 220mg

12. Lemon Garlic Shrimp Pasta

👥 4 | ⏱ 15 min | 🍲 20 min

Ingredients:

- 8 oz whole wheat pasta
- 1/2 lb shrimp, peeled and deveined
- 3 cloves garlic, minced
- 2 tbsp olive oil
- 1 lemon, juiced
- 1/4 cup chopped parsley
- Black pepper to taste

Instructions:

1. Cook pasta according to package instructions. Drain and set aside.
2. In a large pan, heat olive oil over medium heat. Add garlic and sauté for 1 minute.
3. Add shrimp and cook for 4-5 minutes, until pink and fully cooked.
4. Stir in lemon juice and cooked pasta. Toss to combine.
5. Garnish with chopped parsley and serve.

Nutritional Information (per serving):

- Calories: 320
- Protein: 24g
- Carbohydrates: 35g
- Sugars: 2g
- Dietary Fiber: 7g
- Fat: 10g
- Sodium: 140mg
- Potassium: 350mg
- Phosphorus: 220mg

13. Roasted Chicken and Vegetables

👥 4 | ⏱ 20 min | 🍲 45 min

Ingredients:

- 4 chicken thighs, skin removed
- 1 lb baby potatoes, halved
- 1/2 lb carrots, sliced
- 1/2 lb Brussels sprouts, halved
- 2 tbsp olive oil
- 2 cloves garlic, minced
- 1 tsp dried thyme
- Black pepper to taste

Instructions:

1. Preheat oven to 400°F (200°C).

2. In a large bowl, toss chicken thighs, potatoes, carrots, and Brussels sprouts with olive oil, garlic, thyme, and black pepper.
3. Spread the mixture on a baking sheet.
4. Roast for 40-45 minutes, until the chicken is cooked through and the vegetables are tender.

Nutritional Information (per serving):

- Calories: 380
- Protein: 30g
- Carbohydrates: 28g
- Sugars: 7g
- Dietary Fiber: 6g
- Fat: 16g
- Sodium: 130mg
- Potassium: 650mg
- Phosphorus: 280mg

14. Grilled Vegetable Skewers

👥 4 | ⏲ 15 min | 🍲 15 min

Ingredients:

- 1 zucchini, sliced
- 1 yellow squash, sliced
- 1 red bell pepper, cut into chunks
- 1 red onion, cut into chunks
- 1/4 cup olive oil
- 2 tbsp balsamic vinegar
- 1 tsp dried oregano
- Wooden skewers, soaked in water

Instructions:

1. Preheat grill to medium heat.
2. In a large bowl, whisk together olive oil, balsamic vinegar, and oregano.
3. Thread vegetables onto the skewers and brush with the olive oil mixture.
4. Grill the skewers for 10-15 minutes, turning occasionally, until the vegetables are tender and lightly charred.

Nutritional Information (per serving):

- Calories: 120
- Protein: 2g
- Carbohydrates: 10g
- Sugars: 4g
- Dietary Fiber: 3g
- Fat: 9g

- Sodium: 25mg
- Potassium: 300mg
- Phosphorus: 70mg

15. Slow-Cooked Beef Stew

👥 4 | ⏲ 20 min | 🍲 4-6 hours (slow cooker)

Ingredients:

- 1 lb beef stew meat, cubed
- 4 cups low-sodium beef broth
- 2 large carrots, sliced
- 2 large potatoes, diced
- 1 small onion, diced
- 2 cloves garlic, minced
- 1 tsp dried thyme
- 1 bay leaf
- 2 tbsp olive oil

Instructions:

1. In a large pan, heat olive oil over medium heat. Brown the beef on all sides.
2. Transfer beef to a slow cooker. Add carrots, potatoes, onion, garlic, thyme, bay leaf, and beef broth.
3. Cover and cook on low for 4-6 hours, until the beef is tender.
4. Remove bay leaf before serving.

Nutritional Information (per serving):

- Calories: 350
- Protein: 28g
- Carbohydrates: 20g
- Sugars: 4g
- Dietary Fiber: 4g
- Fat: 18g
- Sodium: 130mg
- Potassium: 600mg
- Phosphorus: 220mg

16. Herb-Crusted Tilapia

👥 2 | ⏲ 10 min | 🍲 15 min

Ingredients:

- 2 tilapia fillets
- 1/4 cup breadcrumbs (low-sodium)
- 1 tbsp fresh parsley, chopped

Chapter 6: Dinner Recipes

- 1 tbsp olive oil
- 1 tsp lemon zest
- 1/4 tsp black pepper

Instructions:

1. Preheat oven to 375°F (190°C).
2. Mix breadcrumbs, parsley, olive oil, lemon zest, and black pepper in a small bowl.
3. Coat tilapia fillets with the breadcrumb mixture and place on a baking sheet.
4. Bake for 15 minutes, or until fish is cooked through and crust is golden.

Nutritional Information (per serving):

- Calories: 200
- Protein: 22g
- Carbohydrates: 10g
- Sugars: 1g
- Dietary Fiber: 1g
- Fat: 8g
- Sodium: 50mg
- Potassium: 280mg
- Phosphorus: 200mg

17. Lemon Herb Chicken with Asparagus

👥 2 | ⏱ 10 min | 🍲 20 min

Ingredients:

- 2 chicken breasts, skinless and boneless
- 1 tbsp lemon juice
- 1 tbsp olive oil
- 1/2 tsp dried oregano
- 1/4 tsp garlic powder
- 1/2 bunch asparagus, trimmed

Instructions:

1. Preheat oven to 400°F (200°C).
2. In a bowl, mix lemon juice, olive oil, oregano, and garlic powder.
3. Coat chicken breasts with the mixture and place in a baking dish.
4. Arrange asparagus around the chicken and bake for 20 minutes or until chicken is cooked through.

Nutritional Information (per serving):

- Calories: 220
- Protein: 26g
- Carbohydrates: 5g
- Sugars: 1g
- Dietary Fiber: 2g
- Fat: 10g
- Sodium: 60mg
- Potassium: 350mg
- Phosphorus: 180mg

18. Vegetable Lentil Stir-Fry

👥 2 | ⏱ 15 min | 🍲 15 min

Ingredients:

- 1 cup cooked lentils
- 1/2 cup broccoli florets
- 1/2 cup sliced bell peppers
- 1/2 cup sliced mushrooms
- 1 tbsp olive oil
- 1 tbsp low-sodium soy sauce

Instructions:

1. Heat olive oil in a large skillet over medium heat.
2. Add broccoli, bell peppers, and mushrooms, sautéing for 5-7 minutes.
3. Stir in lentils and soy sauce, cooking for an additional 5 minutes until heated through.

Nutritional Information (per serving):

- Calories: 180
- Protein: 9g
- Carbohydrates: 30g
- Sugars: 5g
- Dietary Fiber: 10g
- Fat: 5g
- Sodium: 120mg
- Potassium: 400mg
- Phosphorus: 150mg

19. Garlic Shrimp with Spinach

👥 2 | ⏱ 10 min | 🍲 10 min

Ingredients:

- 8 large shrimp, peeled and deveined
- 2 cups fresh spinach leaves

- 2 cloves garlic, minced
- 1 tbsp olive oil
- 1/4 tsp red pepper flakes

Instructions:
1. Heat olive oil in a skillet over medium heat.
2. Add garlic and red pepper flakes, sauté for 1 minute.
3. Add shrimp and cook for 2-3 minutes until pink.
4. Stir in spinach and cook until wilted. Serve immediately.

Nutritional Information (per serving):
- Calories: 140
- Protein: 18g
- Carbohydrates: 4g
- Sugars: 1g
- Dietary Fiber: 2g
- Fat: 6g
- Sodium: 130mg
- Potassium: 350mg
- Phosphorus: 150mg

20. Balsamic Glazed Chicken with Roasted Vegetables
👥 2 | ⏱ 15 min | 🍲 25 min

Ingredients:
- 2 chicken breasts, skinless and boneless
- 1/4 cup balsamic vinegar
- 1 tbsp honey
- 1 cup cherry tomatoes
- 1/2 cup sliced zucchini
- 1/2 cup sliced red onion

Instructions:
1. Preheat oven to 375°F (190°C).
2. In a small bowl, mix balsamic vinegar and honey.
3. Place chicken in a baking dish and pour glaze over the top.
4. Add vegetables around the chicken and roast for 25 minutes, or until chicken is cooked through.

Nutritional Information (per serving):
- Calories: 230
- Protein: 26g
- Carbohydrates: 12g
- Sugars: 9g
- Dietary Fiber: 2g
- Fat: 8g
- Sodium: 70mg
- Potassium: 300mg
- Phosphorus: 220mg

21. Herb-Roasted Salmon with Carrots
👥 2 | ⏱ 10 min | 🍲 20 min

Ingredients:
- 2 salmon fillets
- 1 tbsp fresh dill, chopped
- 1/2 lemon, sliced
- 1/2 tsp olive oil
- 1 cup baby carrots

Instructions:
1. Preheat oven to 400°F (200°C).
2. Place salmon on a baking sheet, drizzle with olive oil, and top with dill and lemon slices.
3. Add carrots to the baking sheet and roast for 20 minutes.

Nutritional Information (per serving):
- Calories: 250
- Protein: 24g
- Carbohydrates: 10g
- Sugars: 5g
- Dietary Fiber: 3g
- Fat: 14g
- Sodium: 40mg
- Potassium: 450mg
- Phosphorus: 220mg

22. Turkey and Quinoa Stuffed Bell Peppers
👥 2 | ⏱ 15 min | 🍲 30 min

Ingredients:
- 2 large bell peppers, halved and seeded
- 1/2 cup cooked quinoa
- 1/2 cup ground turkey, cooked
- 1/4 cup diced tomatoes
- 1/4 tsp cumin
- 1/4 tsp garlic powder

Chapter 6: Dinner Recipes

Instructions:

1. Preheat oven to 375°F (190°C).
2. In a bowl, mix quinoa, ground turkey, tomatoes, cumin, and garlic powder.
3. Stuff each bell pepper half with the mixture and place in a baking dish.
4. Bake for 30 minutes, or until peppers are tender.

Nutritional Information (per serving):

- Calories: 210
- Protein: 18g
- Carbohydrates: 18g
- Sugars: 5g
- Dietary Fiber: 4g
- Fat: 8g
- Sodium: 60mg
- Potassium: 350mg
- Phosphorus: 200mg

23. Roasted Eggplant and Tomato Stew

👥 2 | ⏱ 10 min | 🍲 30 min

Ingredients:

- 1 medium eggplant, diced
- 1 cup diced tomatoes
- 1/4 cup chopped onion
- 1 tbsp olive oil
- 1/2 tsp dried basil

Instructions:

1. Preheat oven to 375°F (190°C).
2. Place eggplant, tomatoes, and onion on a baking sheet, drizzle with olive oil and sprinkle with basil.
3. Roast for 30 minutes, stirring halfway through.

Nutritional Information (per serving):

- Calories: 130
- Protein: 2g
- Carbohydrates: 15g
- Sugars: 6g
- Dietary Fiber: 5g
- Fat: 7g
- Sodium: 35mg
- Potassium: 280mg
- Phosphorus: 50mg

24. Chicken and Cauliflower Rice Stir-Fry

👥 2 | ⏱ 15 min | 🍲 10 min

Ingredients:

- 1 cup cooked chicken breast, diced
- 2 cups cauliflower rice
- 1/2 cup snap peas
- 1 tbsp low-sodium soy sauce
- 1 tbsp sesame oil

Instructions:

1. Heat sesame oil in a skillet over medium heat.
2. Add snap peas and sauté for 2 minutes.
3. Stir in cauliflower rice and chicken, cook for 5-7 minutes.
4. Drizzle with soy sauce and serve warm.

Nutritional Information (per serving):

- Calories: 180
- Protein: 18g
- Carbohydrates: 7g
- Sugars: 3g
- Dietary Fiber: 3g
- Fat: 8g
- Sodium: 90mg
- Potassium: 250mg
- Phosphorus: 180mg

25. Coconut Curry with Vegetables

👥 2 | ⏱ 10 min | 🍲 20 min

Ingredients:

- 1 cup coconut milk (unsweetened)
- 1/2 cup diced potatoes
- 1/2 cup diced zucchini
- 1/4 cup chopped onions
- 1 tsp curry powder

Instructions:

1. Heat coconut milk in a saucepan over medium heat.
2. Add potatoes, zucchini, and onions; cook for 15-20 minutes until tender.
3. Stir in curry powder and simmer for 5 minutes. Serve warm.

Nutritional Information (per serving):

- Calories: 190
- Protein: 3g
- Carbohydrates: 22g
- Sugars: 5g
- Dietary Fiber: 4g
- Fat: 11g
- Sodium: 40mg
- Potassium: 280mg
- Phosphorus: 90mg

26. Moroccan-Spiced Chickpea Stew

👥 2 | ⏱ 10 min | 🍽 25 min

Ingredients:

- 1 can (15 oz) chickpeas, rinsed and drained
- 1/2 cup diced tomatoes (no salt added)
- 1/2 cup diced zucchini
- 1/4 cup diced onion
- 1 clove garlic, minced
- 1 tsp ground cumin
- 1/2 tsp ground coriander
- 1 tbsp olive oil
- 1/4 tsp ground cinnamon

Instructions:

1. Heat olive oil in a pot over medium heat. Add onion and garlic, sautéing until fragrant.
2. Add zucchini, chickpeas, tomatoes, cumin, coriander, and cinnamon.
3. Simmer for 20 minutes, until vegetables are tender and flavors meld. Serve hot.

Nutritional Information (per serving):

- Calories: 180
- Protein: 6g
- Carbohydrates: 30g
- Sugars: 7g
- Dietary Fiber: 8g
- Fat: 5g
- Sodium: 30mg
- Potassium: 320mg
- Phosphorus: 100mg

27. Lemon Baked Cod with Asparagus

👥 2 | ⏱ 10 min | 🍽 20 min

Ingredients:

- 2 cod fillets
- 1 tbsp lemon juice
- 1 tbsp olive oil
- 1/2 tsp garlic powder
- 1/4 tsp black pepper
- 1/2 bunch asparagus, trimmed

Instructions:

1. Preheat oven to 375°F (190°C).
2. Place cod fillets in a baking dish, drizzle with lemon juice and olive oil. Sprinkle with garlic powder and black pepper.
3. Arrange asparagus around the fish and bake for 20 minutes or until fish is cooked through. Serve hot.

Nutritional Information (per serving):

- Calories: 200
- Protein: 24g
- Carbohydrates: 6g
- Sugars: 1g
- Dietary Fiber: 3g
- Fat: 8g
- Sodium: 50mg
- Potassium: 350mg
- Phosphorus: 190mg

28. Cauliflower and Spinach Curry

👥 2 | ⏱ 15 min | 🍽 20 min

Ingredients:

- 2 cups cauliflower florets
- 1 cup fresh spinach leaves
- 1/2 cup diced tomatoes
- 1/4 cup chopped onion
- 1 clove garlic, minced
- 1 tbsp curry powder
- 1/2 cup coconut milk (unsweetened)
- 1 tbsp olive oil

Instructions:

1. Heat olive oil in a large skillet over medium heat. Add onion and garlic, sauté until soft.
2. Add cauliflower, tomatoes, and curry powder; cook for 5 minutes.

3. Stir in spinach and coconut milk; simmer for 15 minutes until cauliflower is tender. Serve warm.

Nutritional Information (per serving):

- Calories: 150
- Protein: 4g
- Carbohydrates: 15g
- Sugars: 4g
- Dietary Fiber: 5g
- Fat: 9g
- Sodium: 40mg
- Potassium: 320mg
- Phosphorus: 70mg

29. Baked Chicken with Lemon and Thyme

👥 2 | ⏱ 10 min | 🍲 25 min

Ingredients:

- 2 chicken breasts, skinless and boneless
- 1 tbsp lemon juice
- 1 tsp fresh thyme, chopped
- 1 tbsp olive oil
- 1/4 tsp black pepper
- 1/2 cup cherry tomatoes, halved

Instructions:

1. Preheat oven to 375°F (190°C).
2. Rub chicken breasts with lemon juice, thyme, olive oil, and black pepper.
3. Place chicken in a baking dish and scatter cherry tomatoes around.
4. Bake for 25 minutes or until chicken is cooked through. Serve hot.

Nutritional Information (per serving):

- Calories: 220
- Protein: 28g
- Carbohydrates: 6g
- Sugars: 2g
- Dietary Fiber: 1g
- Fat: 10g
- Sodium: 60mg
- Potassium: 250mg
- Phosphorus: 180mg

30. Eggplant and Tomato Casserole

👥 2 | ⏱ 15 min | 🍲 35 min

Ingredients:

- 1 medium eggplant, sliced
- 1 cup diced tomatoes
- 1/4 cup chopped onion
- 2 tbsp olive oil
- 1/2 tsp dried oregano
- 1/4 tsp garlic powder

Instructions:

1. Preheat oven to 375°F (190°C).
2. Layer eggplant slices in a baking dish. Top with tomatoes, onion, olive oil, oregano, and garlic powder.
3. Cover with foil and bake for 35 minutes or until eggplant is tender. Serve warm.

Nutritional Information (per serving):

- Calories: 140
- Protein: 2g
- Carbohydrates: 14g
- Sugars: 6g
- Dietary Fiber: 5g
- Fat: 9g
- Sodium: 25mg
- Potassium: 280mg
- Phosphorus: 50mg

Dinner Tips and Tricks

Dinner is your opportunity to unwind and nourish your body after a long day. Here are some tips to make your dinner routine easier and more enjoyable:

- **Plan Ahead**: Consider your schedule for the week and plan your dinners in advance. This saves time and reduces stress.
- **Double Up**: Cook extra portions of your dinner recipes so you have leftovers for lunch or another dinner during the week.
- **Flavor Boosters**: Use fresh herbs, lemon juice, and garlic to add flavor without relying on salt. This keeps your meals tasty and kidney-friendly.
- **Enjoy the Process**: Take your time with dinner prep and cooking. Enjoy the process as a way to wind down and relax.

By incorporating these dinner recipes into your routine, you'll end your day with meals that are both satisfying and supportive of your kidney health. Dinner will become a moment of comfort and fulfillment, helping you maintain your renal diet with ease.

Chapter 7: Snack Recipes

Smart Snacking: Fueling Your Day Between Meals

Let's face it—sometimes you just need a little something to tide you over between meals. Snacking can be a crucial part of maintaining your energy levels throughout the day, but when you're on a renal diet, it's important to choose snacks that support your kidney health. The good news? There are plenty of delicious, kidney-friendly snacks that are easy to prepare and will keep your cravings in check.

This chapter is packed with snack ideas that are not only tasty but also low in sodium, potassium, and phosphorus. Whether you're in the mood for something savory or you're craving something sweet, these snacks are designed to fit seamlessly into your renal diet.

So, let's dive into these snack recipes that will keep you energized and satisfied between meals!

28 Kidney-Friendly Snack Recipes

1. Apple Slices with Almond Butter

1 | 5 min | 0 min

Ingredients:

- 1 medium apple, sliced
- 1 tbsp almond butter

Instructions:

1. Slice the apple into thin wedges.
2. Serve with almond butter for dipping.

Nutritional Information (per serving):

- Calories: 160
- Protein: 2g
- Carbohydrates: 22g
- Sugars: 16g
- Dietary Fiber: 4g
- Fat: 8g
- Sodium: 0mg
- Potassium: 200mg
- Phosphorus: 35mg

2. Cucumber and Hummus Bites

2 | 10 min | 0 min

Ingredients:

- 1 cucumber, sliced
- 1/4 cup low-sodium hummus
- 1 tbsp fresh dill, chopped (optional)

Instructions:

1. Slice the cucumber into rounds.
2. Top each cucumber slice with a small dollop of hummus.
3. Garnish with fresh dill if desired.

Nutritional Information (per serving):

- Calories: 60
- Protein: 2g
- Carbohydrates: 8g
- Sugars: 2g
- Dietary Fiber: 2g
- Fat: 3g
- Sodium: 50mg
- Potassium: 150mg
- Phosphorus: 40mg

3. Rice Cakes with Avocado Spread

1 | 5 min | 0 min

Ingredients:

- 2 plain rice cakes
- 1/4 ripe avocado, mashed
- 1 tsp lemon juice
- Black pepper to taste

Instructions:

1. Spread the mashed avocado evenly over the rice cakes.
2. Drizzle with lemon juice and sprinkle with black pepper.

Nutritional Information (per serving):

- Calories: 110
- Protein: 2g
- Carbohydrates: 15g
- Sugars: 0g
- Dietary Fiber: 3g
- Fat: 5g
- Sodium: 5mg
- Potassium: 200mg
- Phosphorus: 45mg

4. Fresh Veggies with Yogurt Dip
👥 2 | ⏲ 10 min | 🍽 0 min

Ingredients:

- 1/2 cup plain Greek yogurt
- 1 tsp lemon juice
- 1 tbsp fresh chives, chopped
- 1/2 cup baby carrots
- 1/2 cup celery sticks
- 1/2 cup sliced bell peppers

Instructions:

1. In a small bowl, mix Greek yogurt, lemon juice, and chives to create the dip.
2. Arrange the vegetables on a plate and serve with the yogurt dip.

Nutritional Information (per serving):

- Calories: 80
- Protein: 5g
- Carbohydrates: 10g
- Sugars: 6g
- Dietary Fiber: 3g
- Fat: 3g
- Sodium: 30mg
- Potassium: 300mg
- Phosphorus: 80mg

5. Homemade Popcorn
👥 2 | ⏲ 5 min | 🍽 5 min

Ingredients:

- 1/4 cup popcorn kernels
- 1 tbsp olive oil
- 1/4 tsp garlic powder (optional)
- 1/4 tsp paprika (optional)

Instructions:

1. Heat olive oil in a large pot over medium heat.
2. Add popcorn kernels and cover with a lid.
3. Shake the pot occasionally until popping slows down.
4. Remove from heat and sprinkle with garlic powder and paprika if desired.

Nutritional Information (per serving):

- Calories: 100
- Protein: 2g
- Carbohydrates: 13g
- Sugars: 0g
- Dietary Fiber: 3g
- Fat: 5g
- Sodium: 0mg
- Potassium: 50mg
- Phosphorus: 40mg

6. Mixed Berries with Mint
👥 2 | ⏲ 5 min | 🍽 0 min

Ingredients:

- 1/2 cup fresh blueberries
- 1/2 cup fresh strawberries, sliced
- 1/2 cup fresh raspberries
- Fresh mint leaves for garnish

Instructions:

1. Combine the berries in a bowl.
2. Garnish with fresh mint leaves and serve.

Nutritional Information (per serving):

- Calories: 60
- Protein: 1g
- Carbohydrates: 15g
- Sugars: 10g
- Dietary Fiber: 5g
- Fat: 0g
- Sodium: 0mg
- Potassium: 150mg
- Phosphorus: 25mg

7. Peanut Butter Banana Bites
👥 1 | ⏱ 5 min | 🍲 0 min

Ingredients:
- 1 banana, sliced
- 1 tbsp natural peanut butter

Instructions:
1. Slice the banana into rounds.
2. Spread a small amount of peanut butter on each banana slice.
3. Stack the slices together to make small sandwiches.

Nutritional Information (per serving):
- Calories: 190
- Protein: 4g
- Carbohydrates: 30g
- Sugars: 14g
- Dietary Fiber: 4g
- Fat: 8g
- Sodium: 2mg
- Potassium: 350mg
- Phosphorus: 55mg

8. Hard-Boiled Egg with Paprika
👥 1 | ⏱ 10 min | 🍲 10 min

Ingredients:
- 1 large egg
- 1/4 tsp paprika
- Black pepper to taste

Instructions:
1. Place the egg in a pot of boiling water and cook for 9-10 minutes.
2. Remove the egg and let it cool. Peel and slice the egg in half.
3. Sprinkle with paprika and black pepper.

Nutritional Information (per serving):
- Calories: 70
- Protein: 6g
- Carbohydrates: 1g
- Sugars: 0g
- Dietary Fiber: 0g
- Fat: 5g
- Sodium: 60mg
- Potassium: 60mg
- Phosphorus: 90mg

9. Almonds and Raisins Mix
👥 1 | ⏱ 2 min | 🍲 0 min

Ingredients:
- 1/4 cup unsalted almonds
- 2 tbsp raisins

Instructions:
1. Combine almonds and raisins in a small bowl.
2. Serve immediately or pack for later.

Nutritional Information (per serving):
- Calories: 180
- Protein: 5g
- Carbohydrates: 18g
- Sugars: 12g
- Dietary Fiber: 4g
- Fat: 10g
- Sodium: 0mg
- Potassium: 200mg
- Phosphorus: 120mg

10. Smoothie with Spinach and Pineapple
👥 1 | ⏱ 5 min | 🍲 0 min

Ingredients:
- 1/2 cup fresh spinach
- 1/2 cup pineapple chunks
- 1/2 banana
- 1/2 cup unsweetened almond milk
- Ice cubes (optional)

Instructions:
1. Combine all ingredients in a blender.
2. Blend until smooth.
3. Serve immediately.

Nutritional Information (per serving):
- Calories: 110
- Protein: 2g
- Carbohydrates: 25g
- Sugars: 15g
- Dietary Fiber: 4g
- Fat: 2g
- Sodium: 60mg

- Potassium: 350mg
- Phosphorus: 55mg

11. Sliced Bell Peppers with Guacamole
👥 1 | ⏱ 5 min | 🍳 0 min

Ingredients:
- 1 red bell pepper, sliced
- 1/4 cup guacamole (low-sodium)

Instructions:
1. Slice the bell pepper into strips.
2. Serve with guacamole for dipping.

Nutritional Information (per serving):
- Calories: 110
- Protein: 2g
- Carbohydrates: 14g
- Sugars: 6g
- Dietary Fiber: 6g
- Fat: 7g
- Sodium: 40mg
- Potassium: 400mg
- Phosphorus: 45mg

12. Yogurt with Honey and Berries
👥 1 | ⏱ 5 min | 🍳 0 min

Ingredients:
- 1/2 cup plain Greek yogurt
- 1 tsp honey
- 1/4 cup mixed berries

Instructions:
1. Spoon Greek yogurt into a bowl.
2. Drizzle with honey and top with mixed berries.
3. Serve immediately.

Nutritional Information (per serving):
- Calories: 120
- Protein: 10g
- Carbohydrates: 18g
- Sugars: 15g
- Dietary Fiber: 2g
- Fat: 2g
- Sodium: 50mg
- Potassium: 200mg
- Phosphorus: 130mg

13. Carrot and Celery Sticks with Peanut Butter
👥 1 | ⏱ 5 min | 🍳 0 min

Ingredients:
- 1 carrot, cut into sticks
- 1 celery stalk, cut into sticks
- 2 tbsp natural peanut butter

Instructions:
1. Arrange the carrot and celery sticks on a plate.
2. Serve with peanut butter for dipping.

Nutritional Information (per serving):
- Calories: 150
- Protein: 5g
- Carbohydrates: 10g
- Sugars: 5g
- Dietary Fiber: 4g
- Fat: 11g
- Sodium: 80mg
- Potassium: 250mg
- Phosphorus: 90mg

14. Baked Kale Chips
👥 2 | ⏱ 5 min | 🍳 15 min

Ingredients:
- 2 cups kale leaves, stems removed
- 1 tbsp olive oil
- 1/4 tsp garlic powder
- Black pepper to taste

Instructions:
1. Preheat oven to 350°F (175°C).
2. Toss kale leaves with olive oil, garlic powder, and black pepper.
3. Spread the kale on a baking sheet in a single layer.
4. Bake for 10-15 minutes, until crisp.

Nutritional Information (per serving):
- Calories: 70
- Protein: 2g
- Carbohydrates: 8g
- Sugars: 1g
- Dietary Fiber: 2g
- Fat: 4g

- Sodium: 30mg
- Potassium: 200mg
- Phosphorus: 30mg

15. Carrot and Hummus Roll-Ups
👥 2 | ⏱ 5 min | 🍳 0 min

Ingredients:
- 2 whole wheat tortillas (low-sodium)
- 1/4 cup hummus (low-sodium)
- 1/2 cup grated carrot
- 1/4 cup chopped spinach

Instructions:
1. Spread hummus on each tortilla.
2. Sprinkle with grated carrot and chopped spinach.
3. Roll up tightly and cut into bite-sized pieces. Serve immediately.

Nutritional Information (per serving):
- Calories: 100
- Protein: 3g
- Carbohydrates: 15g
- Sugars: 2g
- Dietary Fiber: 3g
- Fat: 4g
- Sodium: 100mg
- Potassium: 150mg
- Phosphorus: 40mg

16. Blueberry Almond Bites
👥 4 | ⏱ 5 min | 🍳 0 min

Ingredients:
- 1/2 cup fresh blueberries
- 1/4 cup almonds, chopped
- 1 tbsp honey (optional)

Instructions:
1. Combine blueberries and chopped almonds in a bowl.
2. Drizzle with honey, if desired, and serve immediately.

Nutritional Information (per serving):
- Calories: 70
- Protein: 2g
- Carbohydrates: 9g
- Sugars: 5g
- Dietary Fiber: 2g
- Fat: 3g
- Sodium: 2mg
- Potassium: 70mg
- Phosphorus: 35mg

17. Spiced Apple Chips
👥 4 | ⏱ 10 min | 🍳 2 hours

Ingredients:
- 2 apples, thinly sliced
- 1/2 tsp ground cinnamon

Instructions:
1. Preheat oven to 200°F (95°C).
2. Arrange apple slices on a baking sheet lined with parchment paper.
3. Sprinkle with cinnamon and bake for 2 hours, flipping halfway through.

Nutritional Information (per serving):
- Calories: 40
- Protein: 0g
- Carbohydrates: 11g
- Sugars: 9g
- Dietary Fiber: 2g
- Fat: 0g
- Sodium: 1mg
- Potassium: 70mg
- Phosphorus: 5mg

18. Cherry Tomato and Mozzarella Skewers
👥 4 | ⏱ 5 min | 🍳 0 min

Ingredients:
- 12 cherry tomatoes
- 6 mozzarella balls (low-sodium)
- 1 tbsp balsamic vinegar

Instructions:
1. Thread cherry tomatoes and mozzarella balls onto skewers.
2. Drizzle with balsamic vinegar and serve.

Nutritional Information (per serving):
- Calories: 50
- Protein: 3g

- Carbohydrates: 4g
- Sugars: 2g
- Dietary Fiber: 1g
- Fat: 2g
- Sodium: 40mg
- Potassium: 90mg
- Phosphorus: 50mg

19. Edamame with Lemon Zest
4 | 5 min | 5 min

Ingredients:
- 1 cup edamame (shelled, low-sodium)
- 1 tsp lemon zest
- 1/4 tsp black pepper

Instructions:
1. Steam edamame for 5 minutes or until tender.
2. Toss with lemon zest and black pepper. Serve warm.

Nutritional Information (per serving):
- Calories: 70
- Protein: 5g
- Carbohydrates: 7g
- Sugars: 2g
- Dietary Fiber: 4g
- Fat: 2g
- Sodium: 5mg
- Potassium: 120mg
- Phosphorus: 60mg

20. Frozen Grapes
2 | 5 min (Prep) | 0 min (Freeze 2 hours)

Ingredients:
- 1 cup seedless grapes

Instructions:
1. Wash and dry grapes. Place on a baking sheet and freeze for 2 hours.
2. Serve frozen as a refreshing snack.

Nutritional Information (per serving):
- Calories: 50
- Protein: 0g
- Carbohydrates: 13g
- Sugars: 11g
- Dietary Fiber: 1g

- Fat: 0g
- Sodium: 2mg
- Potassium: 80mg
- Phosphorus: 5mg

21. Roasted Bell Pepper Slices
4 | 10 min | 20 min

Ingredients:
- 2 bell peppers, sliced
- 1 tbsp olive oil
- 1/4 tsp dried oregano

Instructions:
1. Preheat oven to 375°F (190°C).
2. Toss bell pepper slices with olive oil and oregano.
3. Arrange on a baking sheet and roast for 20 minutes. Serve warm or chilled.

Nutritional Information (per serving):
- Calories: 40
- Protein: 1g
- Carbohydrates: 6g
- Sugars: 3g
- Dietary Fiber: 2g
- Fat: 2g
- Sodium: 3mg
- Potassium: 120mg
- Phosphorus: 15mg

22. Banana Oat Bites
4 | 10 min | 15 min

Ingredients:
- 1 ripe banana, mashed
- 1/2 cup rolled oats
- 1/4 cup raisins

Instructions:
1. Preheat oven to 350°F (175°C).
2. Mix mashed banana, oats, and raisins in a bowl.
3. Drop spoonfuls of mixture onto a baking sheet and bake for 15 minutes. Serve warm or cooled.

Nutritional Information (per serving):
- Calories: 70
- Protein: 1g
- Carbohydrates: 15g
- Sugars: 7g

- Dietary Fiber: 2g
- Fat: 1g
- Sodium: 2mg
- Potassium: 90mg
- Phosphorus: 20mg

23. Pear and Cheese Bites
👥 2 | ⏱ 5 min | 🍲 0 min

Ingredients:
- 1 pear, sliced
- 2 oz goat cheese (low-sodium)

Instructions:
1. Top each pear slice with a small amount of goat cheese. Serve immediately.

Nutritional Information (per serving):
- Calories: 80
- Protein: 3g
- Carbohydrates: 12g
- Sugars: 9g
- Dietary Fiber: 2g
- Fat: 3g
- Sodium: 35mg
- Potassium: 80mg
- Phosphorus: 60mg

24. Tomato Basil Bruschetta
👥 4 | ⏱ 10 min | 🍲 5 min

Ingredients:
- 1 cup diced tomatoes
- 1 tbsp fresh basil, chopped
- 1 tsp olive oil
- 4 slices low-sodium whole grain baguette

Instructions:
1. Mix tomatoes, basil, and olive oil in a bowl.
2. Spoon mixture onto baguette slices. Serve immediately.

Nutritional Information (per serving):
- Calories: 60
- Protein: 2g
- Carbohydrates: 10g
- Sugars: 1g
- Dietary Fiber: 2g
- Fat: 2g
- Sodium: 35mg

- Potassium: 60mg
- Phosphorus: 40mg

25. Radish Chips
👥 4 | ⏱ 10 min | 🍲 15 min

Ingredients:
- 1 cup radishes, thinly sliced
- 1 tbsp olive oil
- 1/4 tsp black pepper

Instructions:
1. Preheat oven to 375°F (190°C).
2. Toss radish slices with olive oil and pepper.
3. Spread on a baking sheet and bake for 15 minutes until crisp. Serve immediately.

Nutritional Information (per serving):
- Calories: 30
- Protein: 1g
- Carbohydrates: 5g
- Sugars: 2g
- Dietary Fiber: 2g
- Fat: 1g
- Sodium: 5mg
- Potassium: 90mg
- Phosphorus: 10mg

26. Zucchini Fries
👥 2 | ⏱ 10 min | 🍲 20 min

Ingredients:
- 1 medium zucchini, cut into sticks
- 1/4 cup breadcrumbs (low-sodium)
- 1 tbsp olive oil
- 1/4 tsp paprika

Instructions:
1. Preheat oven to 400°F (200°C).
2. Toss zucchini sticks with olive oil and paprika, then coat with breadcrumbs.
3. Arrange on a baking sheet and bake for 20 minutes until golden. Serve warm.

Nutritional Information (per serving):
- Calories: 90
- Protein: 2g
- Carbohydrates: 13g
- Sugars: 2g
- Dietary Fiber: 2g

- Fat: 4g
- Sodium: 20mg
- Potassium: 150mg
- Phosphorus: 40mg

27. Cucumber Mint Salad
👥 2 | ⏱ 5 min | 🍲 0 min

Ingredients:
- 1 cup cucumber, diced
- 1 tbsp fresh mint, chopped
- 1 tbsp lemon juice

Instructions:
1. Combine cucumber, mint, and lemon juice in a bowl. Serve chilled.

Nutritional Information (per serving):
- Calories: 15
- Protein: 1g
- Carbohydrates: 3g
- Sugars: 1g
- Dietary Fiber: 1g
- Fat: 0g
- Sodium: 2mg
- Potassium: 60mg
- Phosphorus: 5mg

28. Baked Sweet Potato Slices
👥 2 | ⏱ 10 min | 🍲 20 min

Ingredients:
- 1 medium sweet potato, thinly sliced
- 1 tbsp olive oil
- 1/4 tsp cinnamon

Instructions:
1. Preheat oven to 375°F (190°C).
2. Toss sweet potato slices with olive oil and cinnamon.
3. Spread on a baking sheet and bake for 20 minutes until soft and slightly crispy. Serve warm.

Nutritional Information (per serving):
- Calories: 80
- Protein: 1g
- Carbohydrates: 16g
- Sugars: 4g
- Dietary Fiber: 3g
- Fat: 3g
- Sodium: 10mg
- Potassium: 150mg
- Phosphorus: 30mg

Snack Tips and Tricks

Snacking smart is key to maintaining your energy levels and keeping your kidneys happy. The following advice can help you maximize your snack times:

- **Prep in Advance**: Slice fruits and veggies, portion out nuts, and have dips ready to go so you can grab a healthy snack anytime.
- **Mind the Portions**: Even healthy snacks can add up, so be mindful of portion sizes, especially when snacking on high-calorie foods like nuts and peanut butter.
- **Stay Hydrated**: Pair your snacks with a glass of water or herbal tea to keep yourself hydrated throughout the day.
- **Mix It Up**: Keep your snacks varied to avoid boredom. Rotate between different options to enjoy a balanced intake of nutrients.

By incorporating these snack recipes into your daily routine, you'll find it easy to enjoy delicious, kidney-friendly snacks that keep you energized between meals.

Chapter 8: Dessert Recipes

Indulge Without the Guilt: Kidney-Friendly Desserts

Just because you're following a renal diet doesn't mean you have to skip dessert! In fact, enjoying a sweet treat now and then can be an important part of staying motivated and satisfied with your diet. The key is to choose desserts that are low in sodium, potassium, and phosphorus, while still delivering on flavor.

There are many tasty and kidney-friendly dessert recipes in this chapter. These desserts will fulfill your sweet desire without sacrificing the health of your kidneys, whether you're craving something fruity, creamy, or chocolatey.

Let's dive into these indulgent dessert recipes that you can enjoy without the guilt!

30 Kidney-Friendly Dessert Recipes

1. Berry Parfait
2 | 10 min | 0 min

Ingredients:

- 1/2 cup plain Greek yogurt
- 1/2 cup mixed berries (blueberries, strawberries, raspberries)
- 1 tbsp honey
- 1/4 cup low-sugar granola

Instructions:

1. Layer yogurt, berries, and granola in two small glasses.
2. Drizzle with honey.
3. Serve immediately or refrigerate until ready to enjoy.

Nutritional Information (per serving):

- Calories: 160
- Protein: 8g
- Carbohydrates: 25g
- Sugars: 18g
- Dietary Fiber: 4g
- Fat: 3g
- Sodium: 50mg
- Potassium: 200mg
- Phosphorus: 120mg

2. Cinnamon Baked Apples
2 | 10 min | 25 min

Ingredients:

- 2 medium apples, cored
- 2 tsp ground cinnamon
- 1 tbsp honey
- 1/4 cup water

Instructions:

1. Preheat oven to 350°F (175°C).
2. Place the cored apples in a baking dish.
3. Sprinkle the inside of each apple with cinnamon and drizzle with honey.
4. Add water to the bottom of the dish.
5. Bake for 25 minutes, until the apples are tender.

Nutritional Information (per serving):

- Calories: 110
- Protein: 0g
- Carbohydrates: 29g
- Sugars: 25g
- Dietary Fiber: 5g
- Fat: 0g
- Sodium: 0mg
- Potassium: 180mg
- Phosphorus: 15mg

3. Banana Oat Cookies
2 | 10 min | 15 min

Ingredients:

- 1 ripe banana, mashed
- 1/2 cup rolled oats

- 1 tbsp honey
- 1/4 tsp vanilla extract
- 1/4 tsp ground cinnamon

Instructions:

1. Preheat oven to 350°F (175°C).
2. In a bowl, combine mashed banana, oats, honey, vanilla extract, and cinnamon.
3. Drop spoonfuls of the mixture onto a baking sheet lined with parchment paper.
4. Bake for 12-15 minutes, until golden brown.
5. Allow to cool before serving.

Nutritional Information (per serving):

- Calories: 120
- Protein: 2g
- Carbohydrates: 28g
- Sugars: 12g
- Dietary Fiber: 3g
- Fat: 1g
- Sodium: 0mg
- Potassium: 210mg
- Phosphorus: 40mg

4. Lemon Sorbet

👥 2 | ⏱ 5 min | 🍽 0 min (freezing time: 2 hours)

Ingredients:

- 1/2 cup freshly squeezed lemon juice
- 1/2 cup water
- 1/4 cup honey

Instructions:

1. In a bowl, mix lemon juice, water, and honey until well combined.
2. Pour the mixture into a shallow dish and freeze for 2 hours, stirring every 30 minutes until it reaches a sorbet consistency.
3. Serve in small bowls.

Nutritional Information (per serving):

- Calories: 80
- Protein: 0g
- Carbohydrates: 22g
- Sugars: 21g
- Dietary Fiber: 0g
- Fat: 0g
- Sodium: 0mg
- Potassium: 50mg
- Phosphorus: 5mg

5. Chocolate Chia Pudding

👥 2 | ⏱ 10 min | 🍽 0 min (refrigeration time: 2 hours)

Ingredients:

- 1/4 cup chia seeds
- 1 cup unsweetened almond milk
- 1 tbsp unsweetened cocoa powder
- 1 tbsp honey or maple syrup
- 1/2 tsp vanilla extract

Instructions:

1. In a bowl, whisk together almond milk, cocoa powder, honey, and vanilla extract.
2. Stir in chia seeds.
3. Cover and refrigerate for at least 2 hours, or until the pudding thickens.
4. Serve chilled.

Nutritional Information (per serving):

- Calories: 140
- Protein: 3g
- Carbohydrates: 17g
- Sugars: 9g
- Dietary Fiber: 8g
- Fat: 7g
- Sodium: 50mg
- Potassium: 140mg
- Phosphorus: 100mg

6. Baked Pears with Honey

👥 2 | ⏱ 10 min | 🍽 20 min

Ingredients:

- 2 ripe pears, halved and cored
- 1 tbsp honey
- 1/2 tsp ground cinnamon
- 1/4 cup water

Instructions:

1. Preheat oven to 350°F (175°C).
2. Place the pear halves in a baking dish.
3. Drizzle with honey and sprinkle with cinnamon.
4. Add water to the bottom of the dish.
5. Bake for 20 minutes, until the pears are tender.

Nutritional Information (per serving):

- Calories: 100
- Protein: 0g
- Carbohydrates: 27g
- Sugars: 22g
- Dietary Fiber: 4g
- Fat: 0g
- Sodium: 0mg
- Potassium: 150mg
- Phosphorus: 10mg

7. Coconut Macaroons

👥 4 | ⏱ 15 min | 🍲 20 min

Ingredients:

- 2 egg whites
- 1/4 cup honey
- 1 tsp vanilla extract
- 1 1/2 cups unsweetened shredded coconut

Instructions:

1. Preheat oven to 325°F (165°C).
2. In a large bowl, whisk egg whites until frothy.
3. Add honey and vanilla extract, and whisk until combined.
4. Fold in shredded coconut until fully coated.
5. Drop spoonfuls of the mixture onto a baking sheet lined with parchment paper.
6. Bake for 18-20 minutes, until the edges are golden brown.
7. Let cool before serving.

Nutritional Information (per serving):

- Calories: 120
- Protein: 2g
- Carbohydrates: 12g
- Sugars: 10g
- Dietary Fiber: 3g
- Fat: 7g
- Sodium: 20mg
- Potassium: 80mg
- Phosphorus: 30mg

8. Vanilla Almond Milk Pudding

👥 2 | ⏱ 10 min | 🍲 0 min (refrigeration time: 2 hours)

Ingredients:

- 1 cup unsweetened almond milk
- 1 tbsp cornstarch
- 1 tbsp honey or maple syrup

1/2 tsp vanilla extract

Instructions:

1. In a small saucepan, whisk together almond milk and cornstarch over medium heat.
2. Stir continuously until the mixture thickens, about 5 minutes.
3. Remove from heat and stir in honey and vanilla extract.
4. Pour into small bowls and refrigerate for at least 2 hours before serving.

Nutritional Information (per serving):

- Calories: 90
- Protein: 1g
- Carbohydrates: 15g
- Sugars: 12g
- Dietary Fiber: 1g
- Fat: 3g
- Sodium: 20mg
- Potassium: 40mg
- Phosphorus: 10mg

9. Raspberry Sorbet

👥 2 | ⏱ 5 min | 🍲 0 min (freezing time: 2 hours)

Ingredients:

- 1 cup fresh or frozen raspberries
- 1/4 cup water
- 2 tbsp honey

Instructions:

1. In a blender, puree raspberries, water, and honey until smooth.
2. Pour the mixture into a shallow dish and freeze for 2 hours, stirring every 30 minutes until it reaches a sorbet consistency.
3. Serve immediately.

Nutritional Information (per serving):

- Calories: 80
- Protein: 1g
- Carbohydrates: 20g
- Sugars: 18g
- Dietary Fiber: 4g
- Fat: 0g
- Sodium: 0mg
- Potassium: 100mg
- Phosphorus: 10mg

10. Strawberry Banana Ice Cream

👥 2 | ⏱ 5 min | 🍜 0 min (freezing time: 1 hour)

Ingredients:

- 1 banana, sliced and frozen
- 1/2 cup frozen strawberries
- 1/4 cup unsweetened almond milk

Instructions:

1. In a blender, combine frozen banana, strawberries, and almond milk.
2. Blend until smooth and creamy.
3. Pour the mixture into a container and freeze for 1 hour.
4. Scoop into bowls and serve.

Nutritional Information (per serving):

- Calories: 100
- Protein: 1g
- Carbohydrates: 25g
- Sugars: 18g
- Dietary Fiber: 4g
- Fat: 1g
- Sodium: 0mg
- Potassium: 250mg
- Phosphorus: 20mg

11. Peach Crisp

👥 4 | ⏱ 10 min | 🍜 25 min

Ingredients:

- 2 large peaches, sliced
- 1/4 cup rolled oats
- 2 tbsp almond flour
- 1 tbsp honey
- 1 tbsp coconut oil, melted
- 1/2 tsp ground cinnamon

Instructions:

1. Preheat oven to 350°F (175°C).
2. In a baking dish, layer the peach slices.
3. In a small bowl, combine oats, almond flour, honey, coconut oil, and cinnamon.
4. Sprinkle the oat mixture over the peaches.
5. Bake for 20-25 minutes, until the top is golden and the peaches are tender.

Nutritional Information (per serving):

- Calories: 120
- Protein: 2g
- Carbohydrates: 22g
- Sugars: 15g
- Dietary Fiber: 3g
- Fat: 4g
- Sodium: 5mg
- Potassium: 200mg
- Phosphorus: 30mg

12. Blueberry Muffins

👥 6 | ⏱ 15 min | 🍜 25 min

Ingredients:

- 1 cup all-purpose flour
- 1/4 cup almond flour
- 1/2 cup fresh blueberries
- 1/4 cup honey
- 1/4 cup unsweetened applesauce
- 1/4 cup almond milk
- 1 tsp baking powder
- 1/2 tsp vanilla extract

Instructions:

1. Preheat oven to 350°F (175°C).
2. In a large bowl, combine all-purpose flour, almond flour, and baking powder.
3. In a separate bowl, mix honey, applesauce, almond milk, and vanilla extract.
4. Add the wet ingredients to the dry ingredients and stir until just combined.
5. Fold in the blueberries.
6. Spoon the batter into a greased muffin tin, filling each cup about 2/3 full.
7. Bake for 20-25 minutes, until a toothpick inserted into the center comes out clean.

Chapter 8: Dessert Recipes

Nutritional Information (per serving):

- Calories: 140
- Protein: 3g
- Carbohydrates: 25g
- Sugars: 12g
- Dietary Fiber: 2g
- Fat: 4g
- Sodium: 30mg
- Potassium: 70mg
- Phosphorus: 40mg

13. Chocolate-Dipped Strawberries

👥 2 | ⏱ 10 min | 🍽 0 min

Ingredients:

- 1/2 cup fresh strawberries
- 2 oz dark chocolate (70% cocoa or higher), melted

Instructions:

1. Dip each strawberry halfway into the melted chocolate.
2. Place the strawberries on a parchment-lined baking sheet to set.
3. Refrigerate for 10 minutes or until the chocolate hardens.
4. Serve chilled.

Nutritional Information (per serving):

- Calories: 120
- Protein: 1g
- Carbohydrates: 20g
- Sugars: 14g
- Dietary Fiber: 4g
- Fat: 5g
- Sodium: 5mg
- Potassium: 200mg
- Phosphorus: 40mg

14. Vanilla Rice Pudding

👥 2 | ⏱ 10 min | 🍽 25 min

Ingredients:

- 1/2 cup cooked white rice
- 1 cup unsweetened almond milk
- 1 tbsp honey
- 1/2 tsp vanilla extract
- 1/4 tsp ground cinnamon

Instructions:

1. In a medium saucepan, combine cooked rice, almond milk, honey, and vanilla extract.
2. Cook over medium heat, stirring frequently, until the mixture thickens, about 20 minutes.
3. Remove from heat and stir in cinnamon.
4. Serve warm or chilled.

Nutritional Information (per serving):

- Calories: 130
- Protein: 2g
- Carbohydrates: 28g
- Sugars: 13g
- Dietary Fiber: 1g
- Fat: 2g
- Sodium: 50mg
- Potassium: 60mg
- Phosphorus: 40mg

15. Mango Sorbet

👥 2 | ⏱ 5 min | 🍽 0 min (freezing time: 2 hours)

Ingredients:

- 1 cup fresh or frozen mango chunks
- 1/4 cup water
- 1 tbsp honey

Instructions:

1. In a blender, puree mango chunks, water, and honey until smooth.
2. Pour the mixture into a shallow dish and freeze for 2 hours, stirring every 30 minutes until it reaches a sorbet consistency.
3. Serve immediately.

Nutritional Information (per serving):

- Calories: 90
- Protein: 1g
- Carbohydrates: 23g
- Sugars: 20g
- Dietary Fiber: 2g
- Fat: 0g
- Sodium: 0mg
- Potassium: 150mg
- Phosphorus: 10mg

16. Roasted Chickpeas

👥 4 | ⏱ 10 min | 🍽 30 min

Ingredients:

- 1 can (15 oz) chickpeas, rinsed and drained
- 1 tbsp olive oil
- 1/2 tsp smoked paprika
- 1/4 tsp ground cumin
- 1/4 tsp garlic powder

Instructions:

1. Preheat oven to 400°F (200°C).
2. Pat chickpeas dry with a paper towel.
3. In a bowl, toss chickpeas with olive oil, paprika, cumin, and garlic powder.
4. Spread on a baking sheet and roast for 30 minutes, stirring halfway through.

Nutritional Information (per serving):

- Calories: 90
- Protein: 4g
- Carbohydrates: 15g
- Sugars: 1g
- Dietary Fiber: 3g
- Fat: 3g
- Sodium: 20mg
- Potassium: 130mg
- Phosphorus: 50mg

17. Cucumber Slices with Feta and Dill

👥 2 | ⏱ 5 min | 🍽 0 min

Ingredients:

- 1 cucumber, sliced
- 1/4 cup feta cheese (low-sodium)
- 1 tbsp fresh dill, chopped

Instructions:

1. Arrange cucumber slices on a plate.
2. Top with crumbled feta cheese and sprinkle with dill. Serve immediately.

Nutritional Information (per serving):

- Calories: 60
- Protein: 3g
- Carbohydrates: 5g
- Sugars: 2g
- Dietary Fiber: 1g
- Fat: 3g
- Sodium: 90mg
- Potassium: 150mg
- Phosphorus: 50mg

18. Apple Nachos

👥 2 | ⏱ 5 min | 🍽 0 min

Ingredients:

- 1 apple, thinly sliced
- 2 tbsp almond butter
- 1 tbsp raisins
- 1/2 tsp cinnamon

Instructions:

1. Arrange apple slices on a plate.
2. Drizzle with almond butter, sprinkle with raisins and cinnamon. Serve immediately.

Nutritional Information (per serving):

- Calories: 120
- Protein: 2g
- Carbohydrates: 20g
- Sugars: 14g
- Dietary Fiber: 4g
- Fat: 5g
- Sodium: 5mg
- Potassium: 150mg
- Phosphorus: 40mg

19. Veggie Sticks with Hummus

👥 2 | ⏱ 5 min | 🍽 0 min

Ingredients:

- 1/2 cup baby carrots
- 1/2 cup cucumber sticks
- 1/4 cup hummus (low-sodium)

Instructions:

1. Serve veggie sticks with hummus for dipping.

Nutritional Information (per serving):

- Calories: 70
- Protein: 2g
- Carbohydrates: 10g
- Sugars: 3g
- Dietary Fiber: 3g
- Fat: 3g

- Sodium: 35mg
- Potassium: 150mg
- Phosphorus: 40mg

20. Spiced Pumpkin Seeds
👥 4 | ⏱ 5 min | 🍲 20 min

Ingredients:
- 1/2 cup pumpkin seeds
- 1 tsp olive oil
- 1/2 tsp smoked paprika
- 1/4 tsp garlic powder

Instructions:
1. Preheat oven to 350°F (175°C).
2. Toss pumpkin seeds with olive oil, paprika, and garlic powder.
3. Spread on a baking sheet and bake for 20 minutes, stirring halfway.

Nutritional Information (per serving):
- Calories: 90
- Protein: 4g
- Carbohydrates: 3g
- Sugars: 0g
- Dietary Fiber: 1g
- Fat: 7g
- Sodium: 5mg
- Potassium: 80mg
- Phosphorus: 100mg

21. Watermelon and Mint Skewers
👥 2 | ⏱ 5 min | 🍲 0 min

Ingredients:
- 1 cup watermelon cubes
- 10 fresh mint leaves

Instructions:
1. Thread watermelon cubes and mint leaves onto skewers. Serve chilled.

Nutritional Information (per serving):
- Calories: 30
- Protein: 1g
- Carbohydrates: 8g
- Sugars: 6g
- Dietary Fiber: 1g
- Fat: 0g

- Sodium: 2mg
- Potassium: 90mg
- Phosphorus: 10mg

22. Cottage Cheese with Pineapple
👥 2 | ⏱ 5 min | 🍲 0 min

Ingredients:
- 1/2 cup cottage cheese (low-sodium)
- 1/4 cup fresh pineapple chunks

Instructions:
1. Combine cottage cheese and pineapple in a bowl. Serve immediately.

Nutritional Information (per serving):
- Calories: 70
- Protein: 7g
- Carbohydrates: 8g
- Sugars: 6g
- Dietary Fiber: 1g
- Fat: 1g
- Sodium: 90mg
- Potassium: 120mg
- Phosphorus: 100mg

23. Avocado Deviled Eggs
👥 4 | ⏱ 10 min | 🍲 0 min

Ingredients:
- 4 hard-boiled eggs, halved
- 1/2 avocado, mashed
- 1/4 tsp paprika
- 1/2 tsp lemon juice

Instructions:
1. Remove yolks and mix with mashed avocado, paprika, and lemon juice.
2. Spoon mixture back into egg whites. Serve immediately.

Nutritional Information (per serving):
- Calories: 80
- Protein: 4g
- Carbohydrates: 2g
- Sugars: 0g
- Dietary Fiber: 1g
- Fat: 6g
- Sodium: 70mg

- Potassium: 100mg
- Phosphorus: 80mg

24. Pear and Walnut Bites

👥 2 | ⏱ 5 min | 🍽 0 min

Ingredients:

- 1 pear, sliced
- 2 tbsp walnuts, chopped

Instructions:

1. Top each pear slice with chopped walnuts. Serve immediately.

Nutritional Information (per serving):

- Calories: 100
- Protein: 1g
- Carbohydrates: 16g
- Sugars: 10g
- Dietary Fiber: 3g
- Fat: 4g
- Sodium: 0mg
- Potassium: 130mg
- Phosphorus: 30mg

25. Celery Sticks with Almond Butter

👥 2 | ⏱ 5 min | 🍽 0 min

Ingredients:

- 4 celery sticks
- 2 tbsp almond butter

Instructions:

1. Spread almond butter on each celery stick. Serve immediately.

Nutritional Information (per serving):

- Calories: 90
- Protein: 3g
- Carbohydrates: 4g
- Sugars: 1g
- Dietary Fiber: 2g
- Fat: 8g
- Sodium: 10mg
- Potassium: 120mg
- Phosphorus: 40mg

26. Mini Rice Cakes with Tomato and Basil

👥 2 | ⏱ 5 min | 🍽 0 min

Ingredients:

- 6 mini rice cakes
- 1/2 tomato, diced
- 2 fresh basil leaves, chopped

Instructions:

1. Top each rice cake with diced tomato and sprinkle with basil. Serve immediately.

Nutritional Information (per serving):

- Calories: 50
- Protein: 1g
- Carbohydrates: 12g
- Sugars: 1g
- Dietary Fiber: 1g
- Fat: 0g
- Sodium: 5mg
- Potassium: 60mg
- Phosphorus: 10mg

27. Frozen Banana Bites

👥 4 | ⏱ 5 min (Prep) | 🍽 0 min (Freeze 1 hour)

Ingredients:

- 1 banana, sliced
- 2 tbsp dark chocolate chips (low-sodium)

Instructions:

1. Dip banana slices in melted chocolate and place on a parchment-lined tray.
2. Freeze for 1 hour before serving.

Nutritional Information (per serving):

- Calories: 70
- Protein: 1g
- Carbohydrates: 15g
- Sugars: 10g
- Dietary Fiber: 2g
- Fat: 2g
- Sodium: 3mg
- Potassium: 150mg
- Phosphorus: 20mg

Chapter 8: Dessert Recipes

28. Mango Salsa with Lime

👥 4 | ⏱ 10 min | 🍲 0 min

Ingredients:

- 1 mango, diced
- 1/4 red onion, finely chopped
- 1 tbsp lime juice
- 1 tbsp cilantro, chopped

Instructions:

1. Combine all ingredients in a bowl and mix well. Serve chilled.

Nutritional Information (per serving):

- Calories: 40
- Protein: 1g
- Carbohydrates: 10g
- Sugars: 8g
- Dietary Fiber: 1g
- Fat: 0g
- Sodium: 3mg
- Potassium: 75mg
- Phosphorus: 10mg

29. Radish and Cucumber Salad Cups

👥 2 | ⏱ 5 min | 🍲 0 min

Ingredients:

- 1/2 cup sliced radishes
- 1/2 cup cucumber, diced
- 1 tbsp apple cider vinegar

Instructions:

1. Mix radishes, cucumber, and apple cider vinegar in a bowl.
2. Serve in small cups or bowls.

Nutritional Information (per serving):

- Calories: 20
- Protein: 0g
- Carbohydrates: 4g
- Sugars: 2g
- Dietary Fiber: 1g
- Fat: 0g
- Sodium: 5mg
- Potassium: 90mg
- Phosphorus: 10mg

30. Cottage Cheese and Melon Bowl

👥 2 | ⏱ 5 min | 🍲 0 min

Ingredients:

- 1/2 cup cottage cheese (low-sodium)
- 1/2 cup cantaloupe, diced

Instructions:

1. Combine cottage cheese and cantaloupe in a bowl. Serve immediately.

Nutritional Information (per serving):

- Calories: 70
- Protein: 7g
- Carbohydrates: 8g
- Sugars: 6g
- Dietary Fiber: 1g
- Fat: 1g
- Sodium: 90mg
- Potassium: 150mg
- Phosphorus: 100mg

Dessert Tips and Tricks

Dessert can be a satisfying and enjoyable part of your meal plan. Here are some tips to help you enjoy your sweet treats while staying on track with your renal diet:

- **Portion Control**: Even with kidney-friendly ingredients, it's important to keep portions moderate to manage your intake of sugars and carbs.
- **Natural Sweeteners**: Use honey, maple syrup, or fruit to naturally sweeten your desserts, keeping added sugars to a minimum.
- **Make It Ahead**: Prepare desserts like sorbets, puddings, or cookies ahead of time so you always have a healthy treat on hand.
- **Balance Your Day**: If you're planning to enjoy dessert, balance your meals throughout the day to keep your nutrient intake in check.

By incorporating these dessert recipes into your routine, you can enjoy sweet moments while maintaining your kidney health. Dessert doesn't have to be off-limits—it can be a delicious, guilt-free part of your day!

Chapter 9: Kidney-Friendly Drinks, Smoothies, and Juices

Staying Hydrated with Delicious, Kidney-Friendly Options

Staying hydrated is crucial for everyone, but it becomes even more important when you're managing kidney health. The right drinks can help you feel refreshed, energized, and healthy, without putting undue strain on your kidneys. However, not all drinks are suitable—many can be high in sodium, potassium, or phosphorus, which are less than ideal for a renal diet.

This chapter brings together a wide variety of delicious and hydrating recipes that are perfect for those on a kidney-friendly diet. From cooling smoothies and fresh juices to comforting herbal teas and flavored waters, you'll find something to enjoy any time of the day. These drinks are crafted to be low in the key nutrients that can affect kidney health, while still being rich in flavor and nutrition.

Whether you're looking for a quick and nutritious smoothie for breakfast, a refreshing juice to sip on in the afternoon, or a cozy herbal tea to wind down in the evening, this chapter has you covered. Dive into these recipes and discover new ways to stay hydrated and support your kidney health!

Sections:

- **Hydrating Drinks:**
  Cool and refreshing options like infused waters, iced herbal teas, and other beverages designed to keep you hydrated without adding stress to your kidneys.
- **Smoothies and Juices:**
  A selection of nutritious smoothies and juices, perfect for breakfast, a mid-day snack, or any time you need a boost of energy while keeping your diet renal-friendly.

33 Kidney-Friendly Drink Recipes

1. Lemon Mint Water

👥 2 | ⏱ 5 min | 🍳 0 min

Ingredients:

- 1 lemon, sliced
- 1/4 cup fresh mint leaves
- 4 cups water
- Ice cubes

Instructions:

1. In a large pitcher, combine water, lemon slices, and mint leaves.
2. Add ice cubes and stir well.
3. Let it sit for a few minutes to infuse, then serve chilled.

Nutritional Information (per serving):

- Calories: 5
- Protein: 0g
- Carbohydrates: 1g
- Sugars: 0g
- Dietary Fiber: 0g
- Fat: 0g
- Sodium: 0mg
- Potassium: 15mg
- Phosphorus: 0mg

2. Iced Herbal Tea

👥 2 | ⏱ 10 min | 🍳 0 min

Ingredients:

- 2 herbal tea bags (e.g., chamomile, peppermint)

- 4 cups boiling water
- 1 tbsp honey (optional)
- Ice cubes
- Lemon slices for garnish (optional)

Instructions:

1. Steep the tea bags in boiling water for 5 minutes.
2. Remove the tea bags and stir in honey if desired.
3. Let the tea cool to room temperature, then refrigerate until chilled.
4. Serve over ice, garnished with lemon slices if desired.

Nutritional Information (per serving):

- Calories: 20
- Protein: 0g
- Carbohydrates: 5g
- Sugars: 5g
- Dietary Fiber: 0g
- Fat: 0g
- Sodium: 0mg
- Potassium: 0mg
- Phosphorus: 0mg

3. Berry Smoothie

👥 1 | ⏱ 5 min | 🍲 0 min

Ingredients:

- 1/2 cup frozen mixed berries (e.g., strawberries, blueberries, raspberries)
- 1/2 banana
- 1/2 cup unsweetened almond milk
- 1 tbsp ground flaxseed
- 1 tsp honey (optional)

Instructions:

1. Combine all ingredients in a blender.
2. Blend until smooth.
3. Pour into a glass and enjoy.

Nutritional Information (per serving):

- Calories: 130
- Protein: 2g
- Carbohydrates: 25g
- Sugars: 14g
- Dietary Fiber: 6g
- Fat: 4g
- Sodium: 60mg
- Potassium: 220mg
- Phosphorus: 50mg

4. Cucumber Cooler

👥 2 | ⏱ 10 min | 🍲 0 min

Ingredients:

- 1 cucumber, sliced
- 1/4 cup fresh mint leaves
- 1 tbsp lemon juice
- 4 cups water
- Ice cubes

Instructions:

1. In a pitcher, combine water, cucumber slices, mint leaves, and lemon juice.
2. Stir well and add ice cubes.
3. Let it sit for a few minutes to infuse, then serve chilled.

Nutritional Information (per serving):

- Calories: 5
- Protein: 0g
- Carbohydrates: 1g
- Sugars: 0g
- Dietary Fiber: 0g
- Fat: 0g
- Sodium: 0mg
- Potassium: 20mg
- Phosphorus: 0mg

5. Apple Ginger Tea

👥 2 | ⏱ 10 min | 🍲 0 min

Ingredients:

- 1 apple, sliced
- 1-inch piece of fresh ginger, sliced
- 4 cups water
- 1 tsp honey (optional)

Instructions:

1. In a saucepan, bring water to a boil.
2. Add apple slices and ginger, and reduce to a simmer for 10 minutes.
3. Strain the tea into cups and add honey if desired.
4. Serve warm.

Chapter 9: Kidney-Friendly Drinks, Smoothies, and Juices

Nutritional Information (per serving):

- Calories: 15
- Protein: 0g
- Carbohydrates: 4g
- Sugars: 3g
- Dietary Fiber: 0g
- Fat: 0g
- Sodium: 0mg
- Potassium: 30mg
- Phosphorus: 0mg

6. Coconut Water Refresher

👥 2 | ⏱ 5 min | 🍜 0 min

Ingredients:

- 1 cup coconut water (unsweetened)
- 1/2 cup fresh pineapple juice
- 1/4 cup water
- Ice cubes

Instructions:

1. In a pitcher, combine coconut water, pineapple juice, and water.
2. Stir well and pour over ice.
3. Serve chilled.

Nutritional Information (per serving):

- Calories: 40
- Protein: 0g
- Carbohydrates: 10g
- Sugars: 8g
- Dietary Fiber: 0g
- Fat: 0g
- Sodium: 40mg
- Potassium: 150mg
- Phosphorus: 10mg

7. Peach Iced Tea

👥 2 | ⏱ 10 min | 🍜 0 min

Ingredients:

- 2 peach-flavored herbal tea bags
- 4 cups boiling water
- 1 tbsp honey (optional)
- Ice cubes
- Fresh peach slices for garnish (optional)

Instructions:

1. Steep the tea bags in boiling water for 5 minutes.
2. Remove the tea bags and stir in honey if desired.
3. Let the tea cool to room temperature, then refrigerate until chilled.
4. Serve over ice, garnished with fresh peach slices if desired.

Nutritional Information (per serving):

- Calories: 20
- Protein: 0g
- Carbohydrates: 5g
- Sugars: 5g
- Dietary Fiber: 0g
- Fat: 0g
- Sodium: 0mg
- Potassium: 0mg
- Phosphorus: 0mg

8. Cinnamon Apple Water

👥 2 | ⏱ 10 min | 🍜 0 min

Ingredients:

- 1 apple, sliced
- 1 cinnamon stick
- 4 cups water
- Ice cubes

Instructions:

1. In a pitcher, combine water, apple slices, and cinnamon stick.
2. Stir well and add ice cubes.
3. Let it sit for a few minutes to infuse, then serve chilled.

Nutritional Information (per serving):

- Calories: 5
- Protein: 0g
- Carbohydrates: 1g
- Sugars: 0g
- Dietary Fiber: 0g
- Fat: 0g
- Sodium: 0mg
- Potassium: 10mg
- Phosphorus: 0mg

9. Watermelon Cooler
👥 2 | ⏱ 10 min | 🍲 0 min

Ingredients:
- 2 cups watermelon chunks, seeds removed
- 1 tbsp lime juice
- 1 tbsp honey (optional)
- Ice cubes

Instructions:
1. In a blender, puree watermelon chunks until smooth.
2. Stir in lime juice and honey if desired.
3. Serve over ice.

Nutritional Information (per serving):
- Calories: 50
- Protein: 1g
- Carbohydrates: 12g
- Sugars: 10g
- Dietary Fiber: 0g
- Fat: 0g
- Sodium: 0mg
- Potassium: 180mg
- Phosphorus: 10mg

10 Tropical Green Smoothie
👥 1 | ⏱ 5 min | 🍲 0 min

Ingredients:
- 1/2 cup fresh pineapple chunks
- 1/2 cup kale leaves, stems removed
- 1/2 banana
- 1/2 cup unsweetened almond milk
- Ice cubes

Instructions:
1. Combine all ingredients in a blender.
2. Blend until smooth.
3. Serve immediately.

Nutritional Information (per serving):
- Calories: 90
- Protein: 1g
- Carbohydrates: 20g
- Sugars: 15g
- Dietary Fiber: 3g
- Fat: 1g
- Sodium: 20mg
- Potassium: 250mg
- Phosphorus: 30mg

11. Warm Vanilla Almond Milk
👥 1 | ⏱ 5 min | 🍲 5 min

Ingredients:
- 1 cup unsweetened almond milk
- 1/2 tsp vanilla extract
- 1 tsp honey

Instructions:
1. In a small saucepan, heat almond milk over medium heat until warm.
2. Stir in vanilla extract and honey.
3. Serve warm in a mug.

Nutritional Information (per serving):
- Calories: 70
- Protein: 1g
- Carbohydrates: 10g
- Sugars: 8g
- Dietary Fiber: 0g
- Fat: 3g
- Sodium: 50mg
- Potassium: 50mg
- Phosphorus: 10mg

12. Berry Delight Smoothie
👥 1 | ⏱ 5 min | 🍲 0 min

Ingredients:
- 1/2 cup blueberries
- 1/2 cup strawberries
- 1/2 cup unsweetened almond milk
- 1 tsp honey (optional)
- Ice cubes

Instructions:
1. Blend all ingredients until smooth.
2. Serve chilled.

Nutritional Information (per serving):
- Calories: 80
- Protein: 1g
- Carbohydrates: 18g
- Sugars: 12g

- Dietary Fiber: 4g
- Fat: 1g
- Sodium: 30mg
- Potassium: 180mg
- Phosphorus: 20mg

13. Cucumber Mint Cooler
👥 1 | ⏱ 5 min | 🍲 0 min

Ingredients:
- 1/2 cucumber, peeled and chopped
- 1/4 cup fresh mint leaves
- 1/2 cup water
- Ice cubes

Instructions:
1. Combine cucumber, mint, and water in a blender.
2. Blend until smooth.
3. Serve over ice.

Nutritional Information (per serving):
- Calories: 15
- Protein: 0g
- Carbohydrates: 3g
- Sugars: 1g
- Dietary Fiber: 1g
- Fat: 0g
- Sodium: 5mg
- Potassium: 50mg
- Phosphorus: 5mg

14. Apple Ginger Smoothie
👥 1 | ⏱ 5 min | 🍲 0 min

Ingredients:
- 1 apple, peeled and chopped
- 1/2 inch fresh ginger, peeled
- 1/2 cup water
- 1 tsp lemon juice

Instructions:
1. Blend all ingredients until smooth.
2. Serve immediately.

Nutritional Information (per serving):
- Calories: 60
- Protein: 0g
- Carbohydrates: 15g

- Sugars: 12g
- Dietary Fiber: 2g
- Fat: 0g
- Sodium: 1mg
- Potassium: 80mg
- Phosphorus: 10mg

15. Creamy Peach Smoothie
👥 1 | ⏱ 5 min | 🍲 0 min

Ingredients:
- 1/2 cup frozen peach slices
- 1/2 banana
- 1/2 cup unsweetened almond milk
- 1 tsp honey (optional)

Instructions:
1. Blend all ingredients until creamy.
2. Serve chilled.

Nutritional Information (per serving):
- Calories: 85
- Protein: 1g
- Carbohydrates: 20g
- Sugars: 15g
- Dietary Fiber: 3g
- Fat: 1g
- Sodium: 20mg
- Potassium: 200mg
- Phosphorus: 25mg

16. Strawberry Basil Refresher
👥 1 | ⏱ 5 min | 🍲 0 min

Ingredients:
- 1/2 cup strawberries
- 1/4 cup fresh basil leaves
- 1/2 cup water
- Ice cubes

Instructions:
1. Combine all ingredients in a blender.
2. Blend until smooth.
3. Serve over ice.

Nutritional Information (per serving):
- Calories: 30
- Protein: 1g
- Carbohydrates: 7g

- Sugars: 5g
- Dietary Fiber: 2g
- Fat: 0g
- Sodium: 2mg
- Potassium: 100mg
- Phosphorus: 15mg

17. Pineapple Coconut Smoothie

1 | 5 min | 0 min

Ingredients:

- 1/2 cup fresh pineapple chunks
- 1/4 cup unsweetened coconut milk
- 1/4 cup water
- Ice cubes

Instructions:

1. Blend all ingredients until smooth.
2. Serve immediately.

Nutritional Information (per serving):

- Calories: 60
- Protein: 1g
- Carbohydrates: 14g
- Sugars: 11g
- Dietary Fiber: 2g
- Fat: 2g
- Sodium: 15mg
- Potassium: 75mg
- Phosphorus: 10mg

18. Watermelon Lime Cooler

1 | 5 min | 0 min

Ingredients:

- 1 cup watermelon cubes
- 1 tsp lime juice
- 1/4 cup water
- Ice cubes

Instructions:

1. Blend watermelon, lime juice, and water until smooth.
2. Serve over ice.

Nutritional Information (per serving):

- Calories: 35
- Protein: 0g

- Carbohydrates: 8g
- Sugars: 7g
- Dietary Fiber: 1g
- Fat: 0g
- Sodium: 1mg
- Potassium: 60mg
- Phosphorus: 5mg

19. Banana Almond Smoothie

1 | 5 min | 0 min

Ingredients:

- 1/2 banana
- 1 tbsp almond butter
- 1/2 cup unsweetened almond milk
- Ice cubes

Instructions:

1. Blend all ingredients until creamy.
2. Serve immediately.

Nutritional Information (per serving):

- Calories: 120
- Protein: 3g
- Carbohydrates: 15g
- Sugars: 8g
- Dietary Fiber: 3g
- Fat: 5g
- Sodium: 10mg
- Potassium: 180mg
- Phosphorus: 30mg

20. Honeydew Mint Juice

1 | 5 min | 0 min

Ingredients:

- 1/2 cup honeydew melon cubes
- 1/4 cup fresh mint leaves
- 1/2 cup water

Instructions:

1. Blend honeydew and mint leaves with water until smooth.
2. Serve chilled.

Nutritional Information (per serving):

- Calories: 25
- Protein: 0g

- Carbohydrates: 6g
- Sugars: 5g
- Dietary Fiber: 1g
- Fat: 0g
- Sodium: 1mg
- Potassium: 50mg
- Phosphorus: 5mg

21. Papaya Ginger Smoothie

👥 1 | ⏱ 5 min | 🍲 0 min

Ingredients:

- 1/2 cup papaya chunks
- 1/2 inch fresh ginger, peeled
- 1/2 cup water

Instructions:

1. Blend papaya, ginger, and water until smooth.
2. Serve immediately.

Nutritional Information (per serving):

- Calories: 40
- Protein: 0g
- Carbohydrates: 10g
- Sugars: 8g
- Dietary Fiber: 2g
- Fat: 0g
- Sodium: 2mg
- Potassium: 75mg
- Phosphorus: 10mg

22. Kiwi Spinach Smoothie

👥 1 | ⏱ 5 min | 🍲 0 min

Ingredients:

- 1 kiwi, peeled and chopped
- 1/2 cup spinach leaves
- 1/2 cup unsweetened almond milk
- Ice cubes

Instructions:

1. Blend kiwi, spinach, and almond milk until smooth.
2. Serve immediately.

Nutritional Information (per serving):

- Calories: 50
- Protein: 2g
- Carbohydrates: 12g

- Sugars: 7g
- Dietary Fiber: 3g
- Fat: 1g
- Sodium: 15mg
- Potassium: 110mg
- Phosphorus: 20mg

23. Blueberry Coconut Juice

👥 1 | ⏱ 5 min | 🍲 0 min

Ingredients:

- 1/2 cup blueberries
- 1/4 cup unsweetened coconut milk
- 1/4 cup water

Instructions:

1. Blend blueberries, coconut milk, and water until smooth.
2. Serve chilled.

Nutritional Information (per serving):

- Calories: 45
- Protein: 1g
- Carbohydrates: 10g
- Sugars: 7g
- Dietary Fiber: 2g
- Fat: 2g
- Sodium: 5mg
- Potassium: 60mg
- Phosphorus: 10mg

24. Carrot Apple Juice

👥 1 | ⏱ 5 min | 🍲 0 min

Ingredients:

- 1/2 carrot, peeled and chopped
- 1/2 apple, chopped
- 1/4 cup water

Instructions:

1. Blend carrot, apple, and water until smooth.
2. Strain if desired and serve immediately.

Nutritional Information (per serving):

- Calories: 35
- Protein: 1g
- Carbohydrates: 8g
- Sugars: 6g
- Dietary Fiber: 2g

- Fat: 0g
- Sodium: 10mg
- Potassium: 80mg
- Phosphorus: 15mg

25. Mango Lime Smoothie
👥 1 | ⏱ 5 min | 🍳 0 min

Ingredients:
- 1/2 cup mango chunks
- 1/2 tsp lime juice
- 1/2 cup unsweetened almond milk
- Ice cubes

Instructions:
1. Blend all ingredients until smooth.
2. Serve immediately.

Nutritional Information (per serving):
- Calories: 70
- Protein: 1g
- Carbohydrates: 15g
- Sugars: 12g
- Dietary Fiber: 2g
- Fat: 1g
- Sodium: 15mg
- Potassium: 90mg
- Phosphorus: 20mg

26. Pineapple Celery Juice
👥 1 | ⏱ 5 min | 🍳 0 min

Ingredients:
- 1/2 cup pineapple chunks
- 1/2 stalk celery, chopped
- 1/4 cup water

Instructions:
1. Blend pineapple, celery, and water until smooth.
2. Serve over ice.

Nutritional Information (per serving):
- Calories: 40
- Protein: 0g
- Carbohydrates: 10g
- Sugars: 8g
- Dietary Fiber: 1g
- Fat: 0g

- Sodium: 5mg
- Potassium: 55mg
- Phosphorus: 10mg

27. Green Melon Smoothie
👥 1 | ⏱ 5 min | 🍳 0 min

Ingredients:
- 1/2 cup honeydew melon cubes
- 1/2 cup spinach leaves
- 1/2 cup water
- Ice cubes

Instructions:
1. Blend melon, spinach, and water until smooth.
2. Serve chilled.

Nutritional Information (per serving):
- Calories: 35
- Protein: 1g
- Carbohydrates: 8g
- Sugars: 6g
- Dietary Fiber: 2g
- Fat: 0g
- Sodium: 8mg
- Potassium: 90mg
- Phosphorus: 15mg

28. Raspberry Lemonade Smoothie
👥 1 | ⏱ 5 min | 🍳 0 min

Ingredients:
- 1/2 cup raspberries
- 1/2 tsp lemon juice
- 1/2 cup water
- Ice cubes

Instructions:
1. Blend raspberries, lemon juice, and water until smooth.
2. Serve over ice.

Nutritional Information (per serving):
- Calories: 30
- Protein: 1g
- Carbohydrates: 7g
- Sugars: 4g
- Dietary Fiber: 3g
- Fat: 0g

- Sodium: 1mg
- Potassium: 80mg
- Phosphorus: 10mg

29. Orange Carrot Smoothie
👥 1 | ⏱ 5 min | 🍲 0 min

Ingredients:
- 1/2 orange, peeled
- 1/2 carrot, peeled and chopped
- 1/2 cup water
- Ice cubes

Instructions:
1. Blend orange, carrot, and water until smooth.
2. Serve immediately.

Nutritional Information (per serving):
- Calories: 45
- Protein: 1g
- Carbohydrates: 11g
- Sugars: 8g
- Dietary Fiber: 2g
- Fat: 0g
- Sodium: 3mg
- Potassium: 85mg
- Phosphorus: 10mg

30. Pear Vanilla Smoothie
👥 1 | ⏱ 5 min | 🍲 0 min

Ingredients:
- 1/2 pear, chopped
- 1/2 tsp vanilla extract
- 1/2 cup unsweetened almond milk
- Ice cubes

Instructions:
1. Blend pear, vanilla extract, and almond milk until smooth.
2. Serve immediately.

Nutritional Information (per serving):
- Calories: 55
- Protein: 1g
- Carbohydrates: 14g
- Sugars: 9g
- Dietary Fiber: 3g

- Fat: 1g
- Sodium: 5mg
- Potassium: 70mg
- Phosphorus: 15mg

31. Peach Mango Smoothie
👥 1 | ⏱ 5 min | 🍲 0 min

Ingredients:
- 1/2 cup frozen peach slices
- 1/2 cup mango chunks
- 1/2 cup unsweetened coconut water
- Ice cubes

Instructions:
1. Blend all ingredients until smooth.
2. Serve chilled.

Nutritional Information (per serving):
- Calories: 70
- Protein: 1g
- Carbohydrates: 17g
- Sugars: 12g
- Dietary Fiber: 2g
- Fat: 0g
- Sodium: 15mg
- Potassium: 90mg
- Phosphorus: 10mg

32. Grape Apple Juice
👥 1 | ⏱ 5 min | 🍲 0 min

Ingredients:
- 1/2 cup green grapes
- 1/2 apple, chopped
- 1/4 cup water

Instructions:
1. Blend grapes, apple, and water until smooth.
2. Strain if desired and serve immediately.

Nutritional Information (per serving):
- Calories: 60
- Protein: 0g
- Carbohydrates: 15g
- Sugars: 12g
- Dietary Fiber: 2g
- Fat: 0g
- Sodium: 2mg

- Potassium: 80mg
- Phosphorus: 10mg

33. Melon Mint Refresher

👥 1 | ⏱ 5 min | 🍽 0 min

Ingredients:

- 1/2 cup cantaloupe, cubed
- 1/4 cup fresh mint leaves
- 1/4 cup water
- Ice cubes

Instructions:

1. Blend cantaloupe, mint, and water until smooth.
2. Serve over ice.

Nutritional Information (per serving):

- Calories: 30
- Protein: 1g
- Carbohydrates: 8g
- Sugars: 6g
- Dietary Fiber: 1g
- Fat: 0g
- Sodium: 1mg
- Potassium: 60mg
- Phosphorus: 5mg

Drink Tips and Tricks

Hydration is key to maintaining good health, but choosing the right drinks can make all the difference. Here are some tips to help you stay refreshed and hydrated:

- **Infuse Your Water**: Add fruits, herbs, and spices to your water for a refreshing twist without extra calories or sugars.
- **Limit Sugars**: Opt for natural sweeteners like honey in moderation, and focus on drinks that hydrate without adding too much sugar.
- **Stay Cool**: During hot weather, increase your fluid intake with chilled drinks to help regulate your body temperature.
- **Balance Warm and Cool Drinks**: Enjoy warm drinks in the morning or evening to relax, and cool drinks throughout the day to stay refreshed.

By incorporating these kidney-friendly drink recipes into your daily routine, you can enjoy a variety of delicious beverages that support your hydration and kidney health.

Chapter 10: Special Occasions and Holiday Recipes

Enjoying Festivities on a Renal Diet

Holidays and special occasions are a time for celebration, togetherness, and, of course, delicious food. Being on a renal diet doesn't mean you have to miss out on the joy of these festive moments. This chapter provides a collection of kidney-friendly recipes that are perfect for any celebration. Whether it's a family dinner, a festive holiday, or a casual get-together, these recipes will allow you to enjoy tasty dishes while keeping your kidneys in mind.

14 Festive Recipes for Holidays and Celebrations

1. Roast Turkey with Herb Rub

👥 8 | ⏱ 20 min | 🍲 2.5 hours

Ingredients:

- 1 whole turkey (8-10 lbs), thawed
- 2 tbsp olive oil
- 1 tbsp dried rosemary
- 1 tbsp dried thyme
- 1 tbsp dried sage
- 1 tsp black pepper
- 3 garlic cloves, minced
- 1 lemon, halved

Instructions:

1. Preheat oven to 325°F (165°C).
2. Mix olive oil, rosemary, thyme, sage, black pepper, and minced garlic in a bowl.
3. Rub the herb mixture under the skin and over the turkey breast and legs.
4. Squeeze lemon juice over the turkey and place lemon halves inside the cavity.
5. Roast turkey in a roasting pan for 2.5 hours or until internal temperature reaches 165°F (75°C).
6. Let rest for 20 minutes before carving.

Nutritional Information (per serving):

- Calories: 350
- Protein: 45g
- Carbohydrates: 1g
- Sugars: 0g
- Dietary Fiber: 0g
- Fat: 15g
- Sodium: 75mg
- Potassium: 360mg
- Phosphorus: 300mg

2. Sweet Potato Mash (Low-Potassium)

👥 4 | ⏱ 10 min | 🍲 20 min

Ingredients:

- 3 medium sweet potatoes, peeled and cubed
- 2 tbsp unsalted butter
- 1 tbsp honey
- 1/2 tsp ground cinnamon
- 1/4 tsp nutmeg

Instructions:

1. Boil sweet potatoes in water for 15-20 minutes, or until tender.
2. Drain and mash potatoes with butter, honey, cinnamon, and nutmeg until smooth.
3. Serve warm.

Nutritional Information (per serving):

- Calories: 130
- Protein: 2g
- Carbohydrates: 30g
- Sugars: 10g
- Dietary Fiber: 4g
- Fat: 3g

- Sodium: 20mg
- Potassium: 250mg
- Phosphorus: 40mg

3. Green Bean Casserole
👥 6 | ⏱ 15 min | 🍲 30 min

Ingredients:
- 1 lb fresh green beans, trimmed
- 1 cup low-sodium mushroom soup
- 1/2 cup low-sodium bread crumbs
- 1/2 cup unsweetened almond milk
- 1 tbsp olive oil
- 1/4 tsp black pepper
- 1/4 cup onions, thinly sliced

Instructions:
1. Preheat oven to 350°F (175°C).
2. Steam green beans until tender, about 5-7 minutes.
3. In a large bowl, mix mushroom soup, almond milk, olive oil, and black pepper.
4. Combine green beans with the soup mixture and transfer to a baking dish.
5. Top with bread crumbs and onions.
6. Bake for 25-30 minutes until golden and bubbly.

Nutritional Information (per serving):
- Calories: 110
- Protein: 3g
- Carbohydrates: 15g
- Sugars: 2g
- Dietary Fiber: 4g
- Fat: 4g
- Sodium: 45mg
- Potassium: 180mg
- Phosphorus: 30mg

4. Cranberry Sauce (Low-Sugar)
👥 6 | ⏱ 5 min | 🍲 15 min

Ingredients:
- 2 cups fresh cranberries
- 1/2 cup water
- 1/4 cup honey
- 1/2 tsp orange zest

Instructions:
1. In a medium saucepan, combine cranberries, water, and honey.
2. Bring to a boil, then reduce heat and simmer for 10-15 minutes, stirring occasionally.
3. Stir in orange zest and let cool before serving.

Nutritional Information (per serving):
- Calories: 40
- Protein: 0g
- Carbohydrates: 10g
- Sugars: 8g
- Dietary Fiber: 2g
- Fat: 0g
- Sodium: 0mg
- Potassium: 20mg
- Phosphorus: 5mg

5. Apple and Pear Crumble
👥 6 | ⏱ 15 min | 🍲 35 min

Ingredients:
- 3 medium apples, peeled and sliced
- 3 medium pears, peeled and sliced
- 1/4 cup rolled oats
- 2 tbsp almond flour
- 1/4 cup honey
- 1 tbsp unsalted butter, melted
- 1/2 tsp cinnamon

Instructions:
1. Preheat oven to 350°F (175°C).
2. Layer apples and pears in a baking dish.
3. Mix oats, almond flour, honey, butter, and cinnamon in a bowl.
4. Sprinkle the mixture over the fruit.
5. Bake for 30-35 minutes, until fruit is tender and topping is golden.

Nutritional Information (per serving):
- Calories: 130
- Protein: 2g
- Carbohydrates: 28g
- Sugars: 18g
- Dietary Fiber: 4g
- Fat: 3g
- Sodium: 5mg
- Potassium: 120mg
- Phosphorus: 20mg

6. Herb-Crusted Pork Tenderloin

👥 4 | ⏱ 10 min | 🍽 35 min

Ingredients:

- 1 lb pork tenderloin
- 2 tbsp olive oil
- 1 tbsp dried rosemary
- 1 tbsp dried thyme
- 1 tsp garlic powder
- 1/2 tsp black pepper

Instructions:

1. Preheat oven to 375°F (190°C).
2. Rub pork tenderloin with olive oil, rosemary, thyme, garlic powder, and pepper.
3. Place pork in a roasting pan and roast for 30-35 minutes, or until the internal temperature reaches 145°F (63°C).
4. Let rest for 10 minutes before slicing.

Nutritional Information (per serving):

- Calories: 200
- Protein: 30g
- Carbohydrates: 1g
- Sugars: 0g
- Dietary Fiber: 0g
- Fat: 8g
- Sodium: 50mg
- Potassium: 320mg
- Phosphorus: 250mg

7. Pumpkin Pie (Low-Sugar)

👥 8 | ⏱ 20 min | 🍽 45 min

Ingredients:

- 1 1/2 cups pumpkin puree
- 1/2 cup unsweetened almond milk
- 1/4 cup honey
- 1/2 tsp cinnamon
- 1/4 tsp nutmeg
- 1/4 tsp ginger
- 1/4 tsp cloves
- 1 pre-made low-sodium pie crust

Instructions:

1. Preheat oven to 350°F (175°C).
2. In a large bowl, mix pumpkin puree, almond milk, honey, cinnamon, nutmeg, ginger, and cloves.
3. Pour filling into pie crust.
4. Bake for 45 minutes, or until set.
5. Let cool before serving.

Nutritional Information (per serving):

- Calories: 120
- Protein: 2g
- Carbohydrates: 20g
- Sugars: 12g
- Dietary Fiber: 3g
- Fat: 3g
- Sodium: 40mg
- Potassium: 150mg
- Phosphorus: 30mg

8. Garlic Mashed Cauliflower

👥 4 | ⏱ 15 min | 🍽 20 min

Ingredients:

- 1 large head cauliflower, chopped
- 2 tbsp unsalted butter
- 2 garlic cloves, minced
- 1/4 cup unsweetened almond milk
- 1/4 tsp black pepper

Instructions:

1. Steam cauliflower until tender, about 10-15 minutes.
2. In a pan, sauté garlic in butter until fragrant.
3. In a blender or food processor, combine steamed cauliflower, sautéed garlic, almond milk, and pepper. Blend until smooth.
4. Serve warm.

Nutritional Information (per serving):

- Calories: 80
- Protein: 2g
- Carbohydrates: 7g
- Sugars: 2g
- Dietary Fiber: 3g
- Fat: 5g
- Sodium: 15mg
- Potassium: 250mg
- Phosphorus: 20mg

9. Holiday Spiced Pears
👥 4 | ⏱ 10 min | 🍲 25 min

Ingredients:
- 4 ripe pears, halved and cored
- 1 tbsp honey
- 1 tsp cinnamon
- 1/2 tsp nutmeg
- 1/4 tsp allspice

Instructions:
1. Preheat oven to 350°F (175°C).
2. Arrange pear halves in a baking dish.
3. Drizzle with honey and sprinkle with cinnamon, nutmeg, and allspice.
4. Bake for 25 minutes, until pears are tender.
5. Serve warm.

Nutritional Information (per serving):
- Calories: 130
- Protein: 1g
- Carbohydrates: 35g
- Sugars: 28g
- Dietary Fiber: 5g
- Fat: 0g
- Sodium: 2mg
- Potassium: 200mg
- Phosphorus: 20mg

10. Festive Roasted Brussels Sprouts
👥 4 | ⏱ 10 min | 🍲 25 min

Ingredients:
- 1 lb Brussels sprouts, halved
- 2 tbsp olive oil
- 1 tbsp balsamic vinegar
- 1/2 tsp black pepper
- 1/4 cup cranberries

Instructions:
1. Preheat oven to 400°F (200°C).
2. Toss Brussels sprouts with olive oil, balsamic vinegar, and black pepper.
3. Spread on a baking sheet and roast for 20 minutes.
4. Add cranberries and roast for another 5 minutes.

Nutritional Information (per serving):
- Calories: 110
- Protein: 3g
- Carbohydrates: 15g
- Sugars: 6g
- Dietary Fiber: 5g
- Fat: 5g
- Sodium: 10mg
- Potassium: 300mg
- Phosphorus: 50mg

11. Holiday Apple Cider Punch
👥 6 | ⏱ 5 min | 🍲 0 min

Ingredients:
- 4 cups unsweetened apple cider
- 2 cups sparkling water
- 1/2 tsp cinnamon
- 1/4 tsp nutmeg
- Apple slices and cinnamon sticks for garnish

Instructions:
1. In a large pitcher, combine apple cider, sparkling water, cinnamon, and nutmeg.
2. Stir well and refrigerate until chilled.
3. Serve with apple slices and cinnamon sticks for garnish.

Nutritional Information (per serving):
- Calories: 40
- Protein: 0g
- Carbohydrates: 10g
- Sugars: 8g
- Dietary Fiber: 0g
- Fat: 0g
- Sodium: 0mg
- Potassium: 30mg
- Phosphorus: 0mg

12. Light Herb Stuffing
👥 6 | ⏱ 20 min | 🍲 30 min

Ingredients:
- 4 cups cubed low-sodium whole grain bread
- 1/2 cup chopped celery
- 1/2 cup chopped onions
- 1/4 cup unsalted chicken broth
- 2 tbsp olive oil

Chapter 10: Special Occasions and Holiday Recipes

- 1 tbsp fresh parsley, chopped
- 1 tbsp fresh sage, chopped
- 1/2 tsp black pepper

Instructions:

1. Preheat oven to 350°F (175°C).
2. Sauté celery and onions in olive oil until tender.
3. In a large bowl, combine bread cubes, sautéed vegetables, chicken broth, parsley, sage, and pepper.
4. Transfer to a baking dish and bake for 30 minutes, until golden.

Nutritional Information (per serving):

- Calories: 130
- Protein: 4g
- Carbohydrates: 18g
- Sugars: 2g
- Dietary Fiber: 3g
- Fat: 4g
- Sodium: 30mg
- Potassium: 80mg
- Phosphorus: 40mg

13. Carrot and Parsnip Mash

👥 4 | ⏱ 10 min | 🍲 20 min

Ingredients:

- 2 large carrots, peeled and chopped
- 2 large parsnips, peeled and chopped
- 2 tbsp unsalted butter
- 1/4 tsp black pepper

Instructions:

1. Boil carrots and parsnips until tender, about 15-20 minutes.
2. Drain and mash with butter and black pepper.
3. Serve warm.

Nutritional Information (per serving):

- Calories: 70
- Protein: 1g
- Carbohydrates: 12g
- Sugars: 4g
- Dietary Fiber: 4g
- Fat: 2g
- Sodium: 15mg
- Potassium: 200mg
- Phosphorus: 25mg

14. No-Bake Holiday Chocolate Bites

👥 12 | ⏱ 15 min | 🍲 0 min (chill time: 1 hour)

Ingredients:

- 1 cup rolled oats
- 1/2 cup unsweetened cocoa powder
- 1/4 cup honey
- 1/4 cup almond butter
- 1/4 cup unsweetened shredded coconut

Instructions:

1. In a bowl, mix oats, cocoa powder, honey, almond butter, and shredded coconut until well combined.
2. Roll into small balls and place on a baking sheet.
3. Chill in the refrigerator for 1 hour before serving.

Nutritional Information (per serving):

- Calories: 90
- Protein: 2g
- Carbohydrates: 14g
- Sugars: 8g
- Dietary Fiber: 3g
- Fat: 4g
- Sodium: 10mg
- Potassium: 80mg
- Phosphorus: 30mg

Chapter 11: 30-Day Meal Plan

Your Roadmap to a Healthier You

Embarking on a renal diet can feel overwhelming at first, but with a well-structured meal plan, it becomes manageable and even enjoyable. This 30-day meal plan is designed to help you seamlessly integrate kidney-friendly meals into your daily routine. Each day includes breakfast, lunch, dinner, snacks and drink, all using the recipes provided in this book. The meals are balanced, nutritious, and designed to keep your kidney health in mind.

Let's dive into this 30-day meal plan that will guide you through a month of delicious, kidney-friendly eating!

Day	Meal	Recipe	Page
Day 1	Breakfast	Oatmeal with Fresh Berries	PAGE 16
	Lunch	Grilled Chicken Salad with Apple Slices	PAGE 26
	Dinner	Baked Lemon Herb Chicken	PAGE 37
	Snack	Apple Slices with Almond Butter	PAGE 49
	Drink	Lemon Mint Water	PAGE 67
Day 2	Breakfast	Scrambled Egg Whites with Chives	PAGE 19
	Lunch	Tuna Salad Wrap with Cucumber	PAGE 26
	Dinner	Grilled Salmon with Dill Sauce	PAGE 37
	Snack	Cucumber and Hummus Bites	PAGE 49
	Drink	Berry Smoothie	PAGE 68
Day 3	Breakfast	Cinnamon-Spiced Quinoa	PAGE 17
	Lunch	Veggie and Hummus Pita Pocket	PAGE 27
	Dinner	Grilled Salmon with Avocado Salsa	PAGE 38
	Snack	Peanut Butter Banana Bites	PAGE 51
	Drink	Cucumber Cooler	PAGE 68
Day 4	Breakfast	Banana Pancakes	PAGE 17
	Lunch	Quinoa and Black Bean Salad	PAGE 28
	Dinner	Baked Cod with Lemon and Garlic	PAGE 38
	Snack	Carrot and Celery Sticks with Peanut Butter	PAGE 52
	Drink	Peach Iced Tea	PAGE 69
Day 5	Breakfast	Greek Yogurt with Honey and Melon	PAGE 17
	Lunch	Turkey and Avocado Sandwich	PAGE 27
	Dinner	Herb-Crusted Tilapia	PAGE 42
	Snack	Mixed Berries with Mint	PAGE 51
	Drink	Tropical Green Smoothie	PAGE 70
Day 6	Breakfast	Banana Chia Seed Pudding	PAGE 25
	Lunch	Greek Yogurt Chicken Salad	PAGE 35
	Dinner	Eggplant and Tomato Casserole	PAGE 47
	Snack	Banana Oat Bites	PAGE 54
	Drink	Lemon Mint Water	PAGE 67
Day 7	Breakfast	Oatmeal with Fresh Berries	PAGE 16

	Lunch	Spinach and Feta Stuffed Pita	PAGE 33
	Dinner	Garlic Shrimp with Asparagus	PAGE 40
	Snack	Fresh Veggies with Yogurt Dip	PAGE 50
	Drink	Iced Herbal Tea	PAGE 67
Day 8	Breakfast	Cinnamon-Spiced Quinoa	PAGE 17
	Lunch	Veggie Quinoa Pilaf	PAGE 33
	Dinner	Balsamic-Glazed Chicken with Brussels Sprouts	PAGE 40
	Snack	Almond Butter Smoothie	PAGE 29
	Drink	Melon Mint Refresher	PAGE 76
Day 9	Breakfast	Low-Sodium Veggie Omelet	PAGE 16
	Lunch	Mediterranean Chickpea Salad	PAGE 34
	Dinner	Turkey Chili	PAGE 40
	Snack	Sliced Bell Peppers with Guacamole	PAGE 52
	Drink	Grape Apple Juice	PAGE 75
Day 10	Breakfast	Quinoa Porridge with Apples	PAGE 22
	Lunch	Grilled Chicken Salad with Apple Slices	PAGE 26
	Dinner	Grilled Salmon with Dill Sauce	PAGE 37
	Snack	Roasted Bell Pepper Slices	PAGE 54
	Drink	Peach Mango Smoothie	PAGE 75
Day 11	Breakfast	Greek Yogurt with Honey and Melon	PAGE 17
	Lunch	Quinoa and Black Bean Salad	PAGE 28
	Dinner	Baked Lemon Herb Chicken	PAGE 37
	Snack	Frozen Grapes	PAGE 54
	Drink	Iced Herbal Tea	PAGE 67
Day 12	Breakfast	Low-Sodium Veggie Omelet	PAGE 16
	Lunch	Tuna Salad Wrap with Cucumber	PAGE 26
	Dinner	Grilled Chicken Salad with Apple Slices	PAGE 26
	Snack	Peanut Butter Banana Bites	PAGE 51
	Drink	Cucumber Cooler	PAGE 68
Day 13	Breakfast	Banana Pancakes	PAGE 17
	Lunch	Veggie and Hummus Pita Pocket	PAGE 27
	Dinner	Grilled Salmon with Avocado Salsa	PAGE 38
	Snack	Mixed Berries with Mint	PAGE 50
	Drink	Tropical Green Smoothie	PAGE 70
Day 14	Breakfast	Greek Yogurt with Honey and Berries	PAGE 17
	Lunch	Grilled Chicken Salad with Apple Slices	PAGE 26
	Dinner	Herb-Crusted Tilapia	PAGE 42
	Snack	Apple Slices with Almond Butter	PAGE 49
	Drink	Lemon Mint Water	PAGE 67
Day 15	Breakfast	Cinnamon-Spiced Quinoa	PAGE 17
	Lunch	Veggie Quinoa Pilaf	PAGE 33
	Dinner	Grilled Salmon with Dill Sauce	PAGE 37
	Snack	Radish Chips	PAGE 55
	Drink	Iced Herbal Tea	PAGE 67
Day 16	Breakfast	Oatmeal with Fresh Berries	PAGE 16
	Lunch	Tuna Salad Wrap with Cucumber	PAGE 26

	Dinner	Balsamic-Glazed Chicken with Roasted Vegetables	PAGE 44
	Snack	Sliced Bell Peppers with Guacamole	PAGE 52
	Drink	Lemon Mint Water	PAGE 67
Day 17	Breakfast	Low-Sodium Veggie Omelet	PAGE 16
	Lunch	Mediterranean Chickpea Salad	PAGE 34
	Dinner	Garlic Shrimp with Asparagus	PAGE 40
	Snack	Peanut Butter Banana Bites	PAGE 51
	Drink	Peach Mango Smoothie	PAGE 75
Day 18	Breakfast	Banana Chia Seed Pudding	PAGE 25
	Lunch	Grilled Chicken Salad with Apple Slices	PAGE 26
	Dinner	Eggplant and Tomato Casserole	PAGE 47
	Snack	Fresh Veggies with Yogurt Dip	PAGE 50
	Drink	Iced Herbal Tea	PAGE 67
Day 19	Breakfast	Greek Yogurt with Honey and Melon	PAGE 17
	Lunch	Spinach and Feta Stuffed Pita	PAGE 33
	Dinner	Chicken and Cauliflower Rice Stir-Fry	PAGE 45
	Snack	Banana Oat Bites	PAGE 54
	Drink	Grape Apple Juice	PAGE 75
Day 20	Breakfast	Oatmeal with Fresh Berries	PAGE 16
	Lunch	Quinoa and Black Bean Salad	PAGE 28
	Dinner	Roasted Chicken with Lemon and Thyme	PAGE 41
	Snack	Frozen Grapes	PAGE 54
	Drink	Tropical Green Smoothie	PAGE 70
Day 21	Breakfast	Cinnamon-Spiced Quinoa	PAGE 17
	Lunch	Grilled Chicken Salad with Apple Slices	PAGE 26
	Dinner	Baked Lemon Herb Chicken	PAGE 37
	Snack	Mixed Berries with Mint	PAGE 50
	Drink	Lemon Mint Water	PAGE 67
Day 22	Breakfast	Greek Yogurt with Honey and Berries	PAGE 17
	Lunch	Mediterranean Chickpea Salad	PAGE 34
	Dinner	Grilled Salmon with Dill Sauce	PAGE 37
	Snack	Sliced Bell Peppers with Guacamole	PAGE 52
	Drink	Iced Herbal Tea	PAGE 67
Day 23	Breakfast	Oatmeal with Fresh Berries	PAGE 16
	Lunch	Spinach and Feta Stuffed Pita	PAGE 33
	Dinner	Balsamic-Glazed Chicken with Brussels Sprouts	PAGE 40
	Snack	Banana Oat Bites	PAGE 54
	Drink	Melon Mint Refresher	PAGE 76
Day 24	Breakfast	Low-Sodium Veggie Omelet	PAGE 16
	Lunch	Tuna Salad Wrap with Cucumber	PAGE 26
	Dinner	Turkey Chili	PAGE 40
	Snack	Fresh Veggies with Yogurt Dip	PAGE 50
	Drink	Grape Apple Juice	PAGE 75
Day 25	Breakfast	Greek Yogurt with Honey and Melon	PAGE 17
	Lunch	Grilled Chicken Salad with Apple Slices	PAGE 26
	Dinner	Eggplant and Tomato Casserole	PAGE 47

Chapter 11: 30-Day Meal Plan

	Snack	Almond Butter Smoothie	PAGE 19
	Drink	Lemon Mint Water	PAGE 67
Day 26	Breakfast	Banana Pancakes	PAGE 17
	Lunch	Veggie Quinoa Pilaf	PAGE 33
	Dinner	Chicken and Cauliflower Rice Stir-Fry	PAGE 45
	Snack	Fresh Veggies with Yogurt Dip	PAGE 50
	Drink	Iced Herbal Tea	PAGE 67
Day 27	Breakfast	Cinnamon-Spiced Quinoa	PAGE 17
	Lunch	Spinach and Feta Stuffed Pita	PAGE 33
	Dinner	Baked Lemon Herb Chicken	PAGE 43
	Snack	Frozen Grapes	PAGE 54
	Drink	Melon Mint Refresher	PAGE 76
Day 28	Breakfast	Oatmeal with Fresh Berries	PAGE 16
	Lunch	Mediterranean Chickpea Salad	PAGE 34
	Dinner	Garlic Shrimp with Asparagus	PAGE 40
	Snack	Banana Oat Bites	PAGE 54
	Drink	Tropical Green Smoothie	PAGE 70
Day 29	Breakfast	Low-Sodium Veggie Omelet	PAGE 16
	Lunch	Quinoa and Black Bean Salad	PAGE 28
	Dinner	Turkey Chili	PAGE 40
	Snack	Mixed Berries with Mint	PAGE 50
	Drink	Iced Herbal Tea	PAGE 67
Day 30	Breakfast	Greek Yogurt with Honey and Berries	PAGE 17
	Lunch	Grilled Chicken Salad with Apple Slices	PAGE 26
	Dinner	Grilled Salmon with Dill Sauce	PAGE 37
	Snack	Sliced Bell Peppers with Guacamole	PAGE 52
	Drink	Lemon Mint Water	PAGE 67

Tips for Success with the 30-Day Meal Plan

- **Meal Prep**: Spend some time each week prepping ingredients and meals. This will make it easier to stick to the plan and reduce stress during busy days.
- **Stay Flexible**: While the plan provides structure, feel free to swap meals or snacks to suit your preferences and schedule.
- **Stay Hydrated**: Drink plenty of water and kidney-friendly beverages throughout the day to stay hydrated and support your kidney health.
- **Monitor Your Progress**: Keep a journal of your meals, how you feel, and any changes in your health. This can help you stay motivated and track your progress.

By following this 30-day meal plan, you'll not only enjoy a variety of delicious, kidney-friendly meals but also develop healthy habits that support your overall well-being. This plan is designed to be sustainable, ensuring you can maintain your kidney health long-term.

Chapter 12: Practical Tips for Living a Kidney-Friendly Lifestyle

Taking Control of Your Kidney Health

Following a renal diet is just one aspect of managing your kidney health. Incorporating healthy habits into your daily life can significantly improve your overall well-being and help you manage your condition more effectively. This chapter provides practical tips that can help you lead a kidney-friendly lifestyle, keeping your health at the forefront of your choices.

1. Stay Consistent with Your Diet

Consistency is key when it comes to maintaining a renal diet. Here are some tips to help you stay on track:

- **Plan Your Meals**: Use the 30-day meal plan as a guide to organize your weekly meals. Planning ahead reduces stress and helps you make healthier choices.
- **Variety is Essential**: Don't fall into the habit of eating the same foods all the time. Explore new recipes and ingredients to keep your meals exciting and nutritious.
- **Avoid Temptations**: Keep your pantry and fridge stocked with kidney-friendly foods and limit access to items that could jeopardize your health.

2. Hydration: Drink Smart

Staying hydrated is crucial, but it's important to choose the right drinks:

- **Choose Kidney-Friendly Beverages**: Stick to drinks like water, herbal teas, and the kidney-friendly drink recipes provided in this book. Avoid high-sodium, high-potassium, or high-phosphorus beverages.
- **Monitor Fluid Intake**: Depending on your condition, you may need to monitor your fluid intake carefully. Speak with your healthcare provider to determine the right amount for you.
- **Infuse Your Water**: If plain water isn't appealing, try infusing it with fruits, herbs, or cucumbers for a refreshing twist without added sugars or sodium.

3. Regular Physical Activity

Incorporating regular physical activity into your routine can help you manage your kidney health and overall well-being:

- **Choose Low-Impact Exercises**: Activities like walking, swimming, and yoga are gentle on your joints and easy to incorporate into your daily routine.
- **Stay Consistent**: Aim for at least 30 minutes of exercise most days of the week. Consistency is key to reaping the benefits of physical activity.
- **Listen to Your Body**: Pay attention to how your body feels during and after exercise. If you experience any discomfort or unusual symptoms, consult your healthcare provider.

4. Stress Management

Managing stress is vital for maintaining overall health, including kidney health:

- **Practice Mindfulness**: Techniques like meditation, deep breathing, and yoga can help you manage stress and stay centered.
- **Prioritize Sleep**: Ensure you're getting enough rest each night. Quality sleep helps your body recover and manage stress more effectively.
- **Stay Connected**: Maintain a strong support system of family and friends. Sharing your experiences and challenges with others can help alleviate stress and keep you motivated.

5. Keep Track of Your Health

Monitoring your health is essential for managing your kidney condition:

- **Regular Check-Ups**: Keep up with regular appointments with your healthcare provider. Regular check-ups help monitor your kidney function and adjust your treatment plan as needed.
- **Track Your Symptoms**: Keep a journal of any symptoms or changes in how you feel. This information can be valuable when discussing your health with your doctor.
- **Monitor Nutrient Intake**: Pay close attention to your intake of sodium, potassium, phosphorus, and protein. Use the nutritional information provided in this book to guide your choices.

6. Stay Educated

Knowledge is power when it comes to managing your kidney health:

- **Continue Learning**: Stay informed about your condition and the latest dietary recommendations. The more you know, the better equipped you are to make informed decisions about your health.
- **Ask Questions**: Don't hesitate to ask your healthcare provider questions about your treatment or dietary needs. Understanding your condition fully can help you feel more in control.

7. Enjoy Your Food

It's important to enjoy the food you eat, even when following a restricted diet:

- **Experiment with Flavors**: Use herbs, spices, and low-sodium seasonings to enhance the flavor of your meals without adding extra sodium.
- **Focus on Presentation**: Taking the time to present your food in an appealing way can enhance your dining experience and make meals more enjoyable.
- **Savor Each Bite**: Eating mindfully, by savoring each bite and eating slowly, can help you appreciate the flavors and textures of your food.

8. Managing Social Situations

Navigating social situations can be challenging, but it's possible to enjoy yourself while sticking to your diet:

- **Plan Ahead**: If you're attending a social event, eat a small, kidney-friendly snack beforehand to avoid overeating unhealthy options.
- **Bring a Dish**: Offer to bring a dish to share that you know is kidney-friendly. This ensures there's something you can enjoy without worry.
- **Communicate Your Needs**: Don't hesitate to inform the host about your dietary restrictions. Most people are happy to accommodate your needs if they're aware of them.

9. Embrace a Positive Mindset

Your mindset plays a big role in managing your health:

- **Stay Positive**: Focus on the positive aspects of your journey, such as the delicious meals you're able to enjoy and the progress you're making in your health.
- **Set Achievable Goals**: Set small, achievable goals for yourself, such as trying a new recipe each week or increasing your physical activity.
- **Celebrate Your Successes**: Take the time to celebrate your successes, no matter how small they may seem. Each step forward is a victory for your health.

10. Building a Support Network

Having a strong support system can make a big difference in managing your kidney health:

- **Connect with Others**: Join support groups or online communities where you can connect with others who are managing similar conditions.
- **Lean on Friends and Family**: Don't be afraid to ask for help from friends and family. Whether it's emotional support or assistance with meal prep, having people you can rely on is invaluable.
- **Educate Your Loved Ones**: Help your loved ones understand your dietary needs so they can support you more effectively.

By integrating these practical tips into your daily life, you'll find it easier to manage your kidney health while still enjoying a full, vibrant life. Remember, the journey to better health is a marathon, not a sprint, so take it one day at a time and be kind to yourself along the way.

Chapter 13: Dining Out on a Renal Diet

Enjoying Meals Out While Managing Your Kidney Health

Dining out at restaurants can be one of life's greatest pleasures, but when you're on a renal diet, it might feel a bit intimidating. The good news is that you can still enjoy meals out without compromising your health! This chapter will guide you on how to make kidney-friendly choices when dining out, navigate menus like a pro, and even suggest some specific dishes that are perfect for a renal diet.

How to Make Kidney-Friendly Choices at Restaurants

Eating out doesn't have to be stressful or overwhelming. Here are some practical tips to help you make better choices:

- **Communicate Your Needs**: Don't be afraid to tell the waiter about your dietary restrictions. Special requests are usually accommodated by eateries.
- **Avoid High-Sodium Options**: Steer clear of dishes described as "smoked," "cured," "pickled," or "in broth." These tend to be high in sodium.
- **Ask for Modifications**: Request that your food be prepared without added salt, and ask for sauces, dressings, and toppings on the side.
- **Choose Grilled, Baked, or Steamed**: Opt for dishes that are grilled, baked, or steamed instead of fried or sautéed, as these cooking methods typically use less oil and salt.

Navigating Menus: Tips and Tricks

When looking at a menu, it can sometimes be hard to determine which options are the best for your kidney health. Here are some tricks to help you find the right meal:

- **Select Lean Proteins:** Steer clear of highly marinated or sauced proteins and choose lean ones like fish, chicken, or tofu.
- **Focus on Vegetables**: Choose non-starchy vegetables as your side dishes, and ask how they're prepared. Steamed or grilled vegetables are often your best bet.
- **Skip the Bread Basket**: Bread can be surprisingly high in sodium, especially if it's been seasoned or topped with butter. Skip the bread to save on sodium.
- **Be Mindful of Beverages**: Avoid sodas, sweetened teas, or alcohol if you're managing your fluid intake. Opt for water with lemon or herbal tea.

Suggested Restaurant Meals and Modifications

To make dining out even easier, here are some common restaurant dishes and suggestions for modifications to make them more kidney-friendly:

- **Grilled Chicken Salad**: Ask for dressing on the side, skip high-potassium ingredients like tomatoes or avocado, and opt for low-sodium options like lemon juice or olive oil.
- **Baked Fish with Vegetables**: Choose a baked or grilled fish dish with non-starchy vegetables like zucchini, green beans, or peppers. Ask for the dish to be prepared without added salt or heavy sauces.
- **Pasta with Olive Oil and Garlic**: Opt for a plain pasta dish with olive oil, garlic, and herbs instead of a heavy cream or tomato sauce. Add steamed vegetables for extra flavor and nutrition.

- **Egg White Omelet**: For breakfast or brunch, ask for an egg white omelet filled with vegetables like spinach, onions, and bell peppers. Request low-sodium cheese or skip it altogether.
- **Asian Stir-Fry with Tofu**: Choose a vegetable stir-fry with tofu and ask for it to be cooked in minimal oil with low-sodium soy sauce. Avoid dishes labeled as "teriyaki" or "sweet and sour," as these are often high in sugar and sodium.

By using these tips and strategies, dining out can remain a joyful experience, even on a renal diet. Remember, you're not giving up on enjoying delicious food—you're just making choices that support your health!

Chapter 14: Conclusion and Next Steps

Reflecting on Your Journey

Congratulations on reaching the end of this book! This is not the end but the beginning of a new chapter in your journey toward better kidney health. Throughout these pages, you've equipped yourself with essential knowledge about a renal diet, discovered a wide range of delicious recipes, and learned practical strategies to maintain a kidney-friendly lifestyle. Each step you take is a step closer to a healthier, more fulfilling life.

Living with kidney disease requires an ongoing commitment, but with the insights and tools you've gained, you're now empowered to make choices that support your health. Remember that managing your condition is a marathon, not a sprint—take it one day at a time and don't be afraid to seek support whenever you need it.

Celebrate Your Success

It's crucial to acknowledge the progress you've made, no matter how small it may seem. Whether you've mastered a new recipe, stuck to your meal plan for a week, or simply learned more about your condition, these are all victories worth celebrating.

- **Reflect on Your Achievements**: Take a moment to look back on what you've accomplished since starting this journey. Celebrate your successes, and use them as motivation to keep moving forward.
- **Share Your Story**: Consider sharing your experiences with others who are on a similar path. Your story could inspire and motivate someone else who is just beginning their journey.

Continue Your Education

Knowledge is a powerful tool in managing kidney disease. The more you learn, the better equipped you'll be to make informed decisions about your health.

- **Stay Informed**: Continue reading about kidney health, nutrition, and the latest research. Stay up-to-date with new developments and adjust your diet and lifestyle as needed.
- **Ask Questions**: Don't hesitate to reach out to your healthcare provider with any questions or concerns. Understanding your condition fully can help you feel more in control.

Build a Support Network

Having a strong support system can make all the difference in managing your kidney health. Surround yourself with people who understand your challenges and are there to support you.

- **Connect with Others**: Join a support group, either locally or online, to connect with others who understand what you're going through.
- **Lean on Loved Ones**: Don't be afraid to ask for help from friends and family. Whether it's emotional support or assistance with meal prep, having people you can rely on is invaluable.

Keep Setting Goals

Setting goals gives you something to strive for and helps keep you motivated. Whether it's trying new recipes, improving your physical fitness, or maintaining your hydration, goals can keep you on track.

- **Set Achievable Goals**: Start with small, manageable goals that build toward your larger objectives. Celebrate each milestone as you reach it.
- **Reevaluate Regularly**: As you progress, take time to reassess your goals. Adjust them as needed to reflect your current health and lifestyle.

Stay Positive and Persistent

Living with kidney disease can be challenging, but maintaining a positive mindset is key to overcoming obstacles and staying motivated.

- **Focus on the Positive**: Rather than dwelling on restrictions, focus on the positive changes you're making for your health. Embrace the new foods and habits that are improving your well-being.
- **Be Kind to Yourself**: There will be days when sticking to your diet or maintaining healthy habits feels difficult. That's okay. Be patient and compassionate with yourself, and remember that every day is a new opportunity to make progress.

Planning for the Future

Your journey doesn't end here—this is just the foundation for a healthier future. Continue to build on what you've learned and stay proactive in managing your kidney health.

- **Regular Check-Ups**: Keep up with regular appointments with your healthcare provider to monitor your kidney function and overall health.
- **Adapt as Needed**: Your health needs may change over time. Stay flexible and be ready to adjust your diet and lifestyle as necessary.

Encouragement for the Future

This is just the beginning of a lifelong commitment to your health. Here are some final thoughts to keep you inspired and motivated:

- **Stay Curious and Open-Minded**: Continue learning about kidney health, new recipes, and strategies to enhance your well-being. Knowledge is a powerful tool that empowers you to make informed decisions.
- **Celebrate Every Victory**: Whether it's trying a new recipe, sticking to your meal plan, or seeing improvements in your lab results, celebrate each success. These moments of progress are worth acknowledging.
- **Find Joy in the Process**: Focus on the positive changes you're making and find joy in cooking, eating, and living in a way that supports your health. A positive attitude can make all the difference in sustaining long-term success.

Final Words of Support

You are stronger and more capable than you realize. By taking charge of your kidney health, you're not only improving your quality of life but also setting an inspiring example for others. Remember, you're not alone on this journey. Lean on your support network, connect with others who understand your experiences, and never hesitate to seek help when you need it.

Keep moving forward, one step at a time, with confidence and determination. You have the knowledge, tools, and support to navigate this path successfully. Here's to a healthier, happier you!

Thank you for allowing this book to be a part of your journey. May it serve as a source of inspiration, guidance, and encouragement as you continue to make strides toward your health goals.

Glossary of Key Terms

1. Acute Kidney Injury (AKI):

A sudden decrease in kidney function that occurs over hours to days. It can be caused by factors such as dehydration, medications, or severe illness. AKI may be reversible with proper treatment but can also progress to chronic kidney disease if not managed promptly.

2. Albuminuria:

The presence of albumin (a type of protein) in the urine, which can be an early sign of kidney damage. Healthy kidneys do not allow albumin to pass into the urine, so its presence indicates that the kidneys are not functioning properly.

3. Anemia:

A condition in which the body does not have enough red blood cells or hemoglobin to carry adequate oxygen to tissues, often occurring in people with chronic kidney disease due to reduced production of erythropoietin, a hormone produced by the kidneys.

4. Blood Urea Nitrogen (BUN):

A test that measures the amount of nitrogen in the blood in the form of urea, a waste product formed from the breakdown of protein. High levels of BUN may indicate impaired kidney function or dehydration.

5. Chronic Kidney Disease (CKD):

A long-term condition characterized by gradual loss of kidney function over time. CKD is divided into five stages, with Stage 1 being mild damage and Stage 5 being kidney failure requiring dialysis or transplantation.

6. Creatinine:

A waste product produced by muscles from the breakdown of creatine, which is removed from the blood by the kidneys. Elevated creatinine levels in the blood can indicate impaired kidney function.

7. Dialysis:

A medical treatment used to remove waste products and excess fluids from the blood when the kidneys are no longer able to do so. There are two main types: hemodialysis (performed using a machine) and peritoneal dialysis (performed using the lining of the abdomen as a filter).

8. Electrolytes:

Minerals in the blood and body fluids, such as sodium, potassium, and phosphorus, that are essential for maintaining proper body function, including muscle contraction and nerve signaling. Kidney disease can cause imbalances in electrolyte levels.

9. Erythropoietin (EPO):

A hormone produced by the kidneys that stimulates the production of red blood cells in the bone marrow. In people with kidney disease, EPO production may decrease, leading to anemia.

10. Estimated Glomerular Filtration Rate (eGFR):

A calculation used to assess kidney function by estimating the rate at which the kidneys filter waste products from the blood. It is based on blood creatinine levels, age, sex, and other factors.

11. Glomerulus:

A network of tiny blood vessels (capillaries) in the kidneys where blood filtration begins. The glomerulus allows water, salts, and waste products to pass through while retaining larger molecules like proteins and blood cells.

12. Hematuria:

The presence of blood in the urine, which can be a sign of kidney disease, infection, or injury. Hematuria may be visible to the naked eye (gross hematuria) or detected only under a microscope (microscopic hematuria).

13. Hyperkalemia:

A condition characterized by elevated potassium levels in the blood, which can be dangerous and cause symptoms like muscle weakness, fatigue, and heart rhythm problems. People with kidney disease are at a higher risk of hyperkalemia due to reduced ability to excrete potassium.

14. Hypertension:

Also known as high blood pressure, hypertension is a common condition in which the force of blood against the artery walls is consistently too high. It is both a cause and a complication of kidney disease.

15. Nephron:

The functional unit of the kidney, consisting of a glomerulus and a tubule, where blood filtration, waste removal, and water balance occur. Each kidney contains about a million nephrons.

16. Phosphorus:

A mineral found in many foods, essential for healthy bones and teeth. In kidney disease, phosphorus can build up in the blood, leading to weakened bones, heart disease, and other complications.

17. Polycystic Kidney Disease (PKD):

A genetic disorder characterized by the growth of numerous cysts in the kidneys, which can lead to kidney enlargement and loss of function over time.

18. Proteinuria:

The presence of an abnormal amount of protein in the urine, which is often an early sign of kidney disease. It can occur due to damage to the glomeruli, allowing protein to leak into the urine.

19. Renal Diet:

A diet designed to manage the intake of certain nutrients (such as sodium, potassium, and phosphorus) to reduce the burden on the kidneys and prevent further damage. It often includes low-sodium, low-potassium, and low-phosphorus foods.

20. Sodium:

An essential mineral found in salt, necessary for fluid balance, nerve function, and muscle contraction. In people with kidney disease, excess sodium can lead to fluid retention, high blood pressure, and worsening kidney function.

21. Stage 5 CKD (End-Stage Renal Disease or ESRD):

The final stage of chronic kidney disease, in which the kidneys have lost nearly all their function (eGFR below 15 mL/min). At this stage, dialysis or a kidney transplant is required to sustain life.

22. Uremia:

A condition in which urea and other waste products build up in the blood due to impaired kidney function. Symptoms of uremia include nausea, vomiting, fatigue, confusion, and can be life-threatening if untreated.

23. Urinary Tract Infection (UTI):

An infection that occurs in any part of the urinary system, including the kidneys, ureters, bladder, or urethra. UTIs can sometimes lead to more serious kidney infections if not treated promptly.

24. Vitamin D:

A vitamin that helps regulate calcium and phosphorus levels in the blood, promoting bone health. Kidneys help convert vitamin D into its active form; kidney disease can impair this function, leading to deficiencies.

25. Water Retention:

Also known as edema, water retention occurs when the body holds onto excess fluids, often causing swelling in the legs, feet, or hands. This can be a common complication in people with kidney disease.

Get your free bonuses

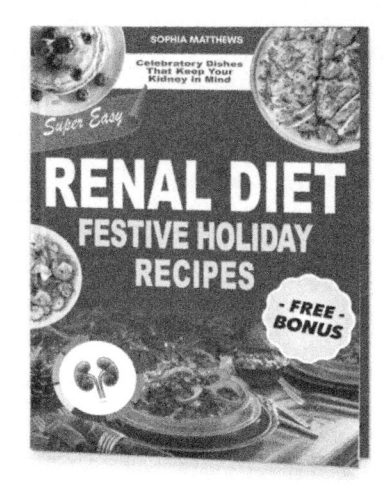

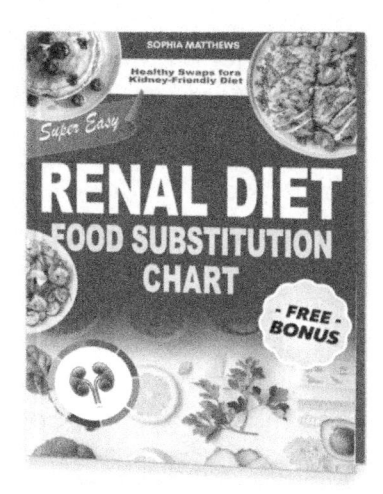

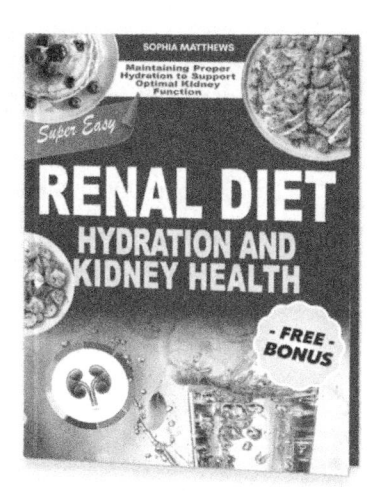

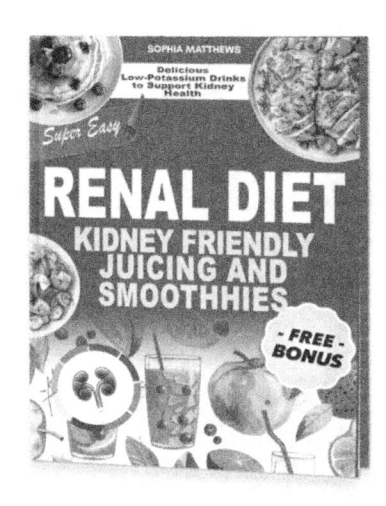

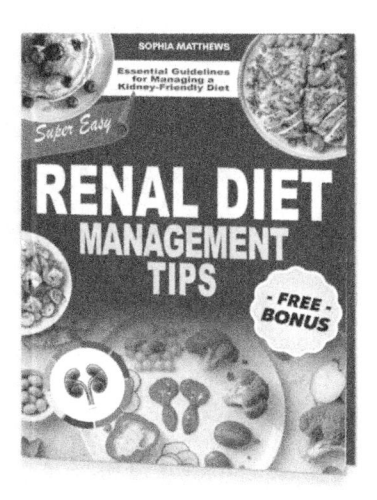

Discover a wealth of exclusive resources to enhance your kidney health journey and optimize your well-being!

Scan the QR code now to download them for free and take the first step toward a healthier, kidney-friendly lifestyle!

Did you enjoy this book?

I hope this collection of kidney-friendly, nutrient-packed recipes has inspired and energized your journey toward better kidney health! Your feedback is incredibly valuable to me.

Your positive review not only helps others discover the book, but it also strengthens our growing community of kidney health enthusiasts.
Leaving a review is simple just scan the QR code below to share your favorite parts through a quick feedback form!
And if you have suggestions or ideas, I'd love to hear them.
Your input is essential in helping me provide even better resources.
Thank you so much for your support!

All rights reserved No portion of " Renal Diet Cookbook for Beginners " may be replicated or disseminated in any form without written consent from the copyright owner, Sophia Matthews, barring some permitted uses under copyright law.
©2024 Sophia Matthews.

Printed in Dunstable, United Kingdom